If there are 5 billion people in the world, then it is likely that 3 billion have pelvic instability because they suffer BACK and other musculo-skeletal pains. Most observant practitioners of whatever medical persuasion will agree that the greater majority of their patients have comparative leg-length discrepancy, i.e. one leg longer than the other, including themselves:

> *Leg length discrepancy is a symptom of pelvic distortion.*

In truth, the average is one in a hundred people exhibiting true comparative leg-length difference once **Pelvic Correction** has been administered.

Perhaps the **Creator** wondrously made us perfect as long as we inherited 'a full pack of cards' so to speak. The trouble is: so many adverse factors intercede during our lifetime that imperfections develop. These cause a series of pathological weaknesses: **pelvic instability being one of them.** Read: **Some Reasons Why We Suffer Pelvic Instability** on Page 9.

The Alexander Barrie System of Pelvic Correction™ (ABSPC) outlined in this manual allows you to be empowered and in control, pain-wise, over the health of your **back, shoulder, upper arm, neck, knee and more,** by teaching you how to keep the integrity of the pelvis.

In addition, certain health conditions such as with headache and digestive problems may well resolve.

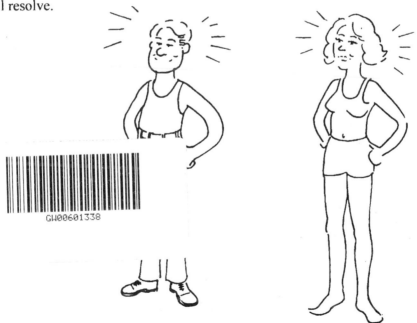

GW00601338

Correct Your Pelvis and Heal Your Back-pain

The self-help manual for alleviating back-pain and other musculo-skeletal aches and pains

The Alexander Barrie System of Pelvic Correction™

By: Alexander Barrie

Published by: Alexander Barrie

Dedicated To: The Creator's Splendour

Alexander Barrie. Harrow. United Kingdom. Published 2005.
© Alexander Barrie 2005. All Rights Reserved.

ISBN   0-9549755-0-2

The Alexander Barrie System of Pelvic Correction ™

For additional information and to read on Testimonials:
WEBSITE: www.alexalign.com

For 2-Day or 1-Day workshops on Pelvic Correction
Contact:
EMAIL: abspc@btinternet.com

SOME HORRIFYING FACTS

Back-pain is a serious worldwide problem as well as being a coňundrum to all those who treat patients with back-pain, ostensibly! In the developed world, back-pain has reached epidemic proportions. It causes great suffering and fearfulness to the individual and represents a major drain on our Economies and Health Budgets. See Statistics from Page 70.

The far-reaching impact of back-pain must not be underestimated. Statistics from the National Institute of Health indicate that 75-80% of all people suffer back-pain at some time during their lives. It ranges from dull deep annoying pain to severe disabling pain - enough to prevent you from enjoying your normal life.

This phenomenon is the same worldwide. Millions of people, an astonishing number, suffer from it at some time if not all the time, and so you are not alone!

The doctors suggest many causes for the existence of back-pain. These may cover factors such as with strenuous activity, fracture, degeneration of spinal vertebrae, infection, obesity, poor muscle tone, sprain, sports injuries, joint problems, disease, smoking and others. Even with today's advanced technology, the **exact** cause can be found only in very few cases.

We place too much pressure on our backs. This is unavoidable. We, as homo-sapien, have done so, since we started to walk upright. **However, we can help ourselves – if we learn to control the stability of the pelvis:**

Alexander Barrie's work as Back-pain Consultant is at the cutting-edge of back-pain cure. For more than a decade, he has treated more than 11,000 people from all 'walks of life' and from all over the world.

His unique treatment System – The Alexander Barrie System of Pelvic Correction™ - produces dramatic results, with many of his patients experiencing 'life changing' and permanent relief from back-pain and other musculo-skeletal problems. (Read Testimonials pages 79 to 82. Biographical Note page 85)

The great success of Alexander Barrie's System may be attributed to a fundamental observation he made early in his therapeutic career – and one that changed the course of his professional life.

Though patients presented with a variety of aches and pains, acute and chronic, closer examination revealed that almost all of them (over 98%) shared a common characteristic:
<u>PELVIC MISALIGNMENT & LEG LENGTH DISCREPANCY</u>

Read from Chapter 2: Mechanics & Dysfunctions of Pelvis & Legs

CONTENTS

Written by, and Pelvic Correction System created by
Alexander Barrie *MRSS. RCST. ABSPC*
Harrow, England.

Illustrations by Michael D. Zeffert *AD*

Dedicated to: The Creator's Splendour

Chapter One

THE SELF-HELP MANUAL OF PELVIC CORRECTION FOR CONTROL & ELIMINATION OF BACK-PAIN AND MORE

The reason for this elementary manual is to bring to the attention of everyone, the truth that 85% of them [**you**] do not have to suffer back, shoulder, neck, and knee pain and more. You have the power **now** and the gaining of knowledge to heal yourself.

> *Provided an X-ray or Scan diagnosis does not reveal: A spinal tumour (on bone or brainstem); tuberculosis of vertebra/disc; osteoarthritis causing outgrowths [spurs] on vertebrae [exostosis]; osteoporosis, causing a dysfunctional (crumbling) vertebra, also because of spinal compression. Spondylolisthesis (the slipping forward of a vertebra over the one below it); herniated disc; kidney infection; intrapelvic mass (polyps, tumours) occluding various vessels and, other not so common conditions; then you need not endure back-pain etc., It is likely that no more than 20% of mankind suffers from any one of the conditions outlined above.*

There are a number of groups of physicians both orthodox and alternative in their medical approaches, that know: the **stability of the pelvis underlies the health of the spine.** Many Osteopaths and Chiropractors as individuals know this. Many Russian, American and Japanese Physicians **especially** know this as well.

Some of these professionals have systemised their own way of dealing with the spine successfully **via the pelvis**. However, until the publication of this self-help manual there was no unifying corpus of knowledge and skill all these disparate groups and individuals could employ.

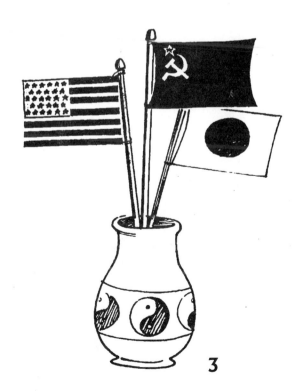

BEFORE YOU DO ANYTHING:

I suggest you begin with the **'Regulator' Technique** on the next page, followed by the 'Thumb Drive' Technique and then the 'Lumbar Rub' Technique. These three, practiced diligently should correct the pelvis regardless of the type of problem your pelvis suffers. Indeed, you could say that they are fail-safe as long as instructions are adhered to, and especially so, if Part A of the 'Regulator' is performed at absolute maximum strength.

The reason why these techniques have been chosen from the start is because they should satisfy the desire of the reader to get himself out of aches and pains, immediately if possible.

These techniques should meet the challenge for pelvic re-alignment; even so, you should visit a chiropractor or osteopath for treatments (although this is not essential) to assist re-alignment of your spine. You will enjoy success with these types of treatment, as you yourself are the one looking after your own pelvis – so difficult to do so by the 'professionals'

The reason for success in pain relief now, is, because, you are the one re-adjusting your pelvis daily. Pelvic instability, so commonplace, underlies virtually all back disorders.

Following the application of these techniques the remainder of this manual may be studied, and other techniques practiced (though optional) to make more concrete and permanent the good changes that have taken place for most of you.

In addition, you will learn why you suffer pain, at all! Of course, there are those people whose musculo-skeletal problems are more complicated, and beyond the scope of this manual. These people ideally need to visit my clinic in London, England.

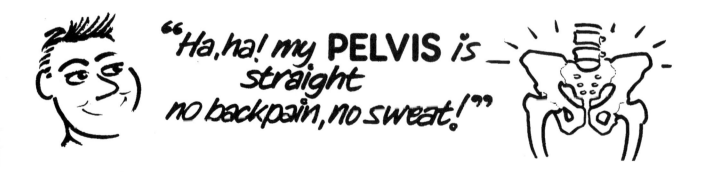

"Ha, ha! my PELVIS is straight no backpain, no sweat!"

THE REGULATOR TECHNIQUE

The following technique is probably the most successful of all Pelvic Correction procedures. It cuts through the absolute requirement to know what type of dysfunction your pelvis suffers. In execution, it should be repeated at least once. It is essential to apply 100% of your full strength when performing PART A, but not to the point of strain. **Execute this technique at least 3 times a day** and more if possible. As back-up to this technique, I recommend that you practice also the techniques on both pages 7 and 38, at least once a day.

Part A:

- Lie down face upwards (supine), arms resting on chest or placed behind head
- Draw both knees upwards, feet together and fairly close to buttocks
- You may use a thin rolled-up telephone book or the like, it, held by sticky tape or elastic bands. Place this between your knees. Any object will suffice as long as it is A4 length (9 to 12 inches)
- Take a breath, hold this breath in, for a count of up to 16 (2 counts per second) and simultaneously try to bring both knees together at 100% strength (adduction). The object between your knees is resisting them being brought together, quite rightly. You may hear a click or clunk or a tearing sound – this is good
- Holding your breath enables you to keep your strength with this exertion. In this first Part A, your sacro-iliac joints are fractionally moved apart to allow the specialised and distorted ligaments holding these pelvic components together, to reset, and the pelvis re-aligns as a result

Part B:

- Bring both knees together
- Wrap around both knees a belt or tie of some kind
- Take a breath and hold this breath exactly as indicated above simultaneously trying to separate both knees (abduction) at strength, though this need not be as strong as that required in Part A
- Repeat Part A and Part B once more
- Get up and walk around to move blood through the system

You may apply this technique when sitting, as long as your torso is upright. This means you may perform it anywhere at any time – and this is required! Simply apply the self same instructions indicated above for your sitting mode, though sitting on the very outer edge of the seat is required. Of course, the laying-down version is best, but you cannot find a place during the day when 'out and about' to lie-down, and so the sitting version is the next best thing.

5

THE 'REGULATOR' TECHNIQUE: ILLUSTRATION 1.
(Follow-up this technique with: <u>Thumb Drive</u> page 7 & <u>Lumbar Rub</u> page 38)

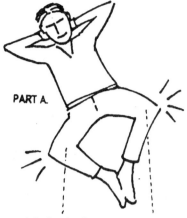

PART A.

A helper's forearm, or an object, acting as a wedge here, to keep knees apart. Keep feet together.

A helper's hands, or belt wrapped around and underneath knees here, keeps knees together. Keep feet together.

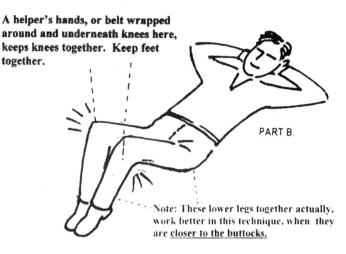

PART B.

Note: These lower legs together actually, work better in this technique, when they are <u>closer to the buttocks</u>.

At the time of updating this manual (early 2005), the prototype 'Pelvic Corrector' device called: BACKCHAMP® has been created to allow easy execution of the 'Regulator' Technique. This device, brilliantly designed by Jeffrey James, London, and taken from original drawings by Alexander Barrie, saves the tiresome use of the 'book and the belt' to enable the 'Regulator' Technique to be carried-out.

It will be seen from some of the Testimonials in this manual, page 79 how successful the application of the BACKCHAMP® has become.

Within the first 6 months of 2005, it is assumed there will be a Website specific to the BACKCHAMP® as the intention is: to make the device more appealing, using different materials and packaged for world-wide availability.

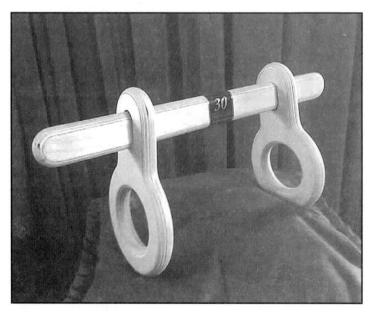

For the moment, this prototype is available only from the Alexanderbase. See Website: www.alexalign.com

Read on
BACKCHAMP®
Page 8

Please read:
ESSENTIAL NOTES
ABSOLUTE
At the very end of
this manual P.84

'THUMB DRIVE' TECHNIQUE

The following technique is very effective to make more concrete the good results of the application of the technique on the previous page. However, the 'Thumb Drive' is very efficacious in its own right, in that it can also re-align the pelvis. There are caveats to this: which are: 1. A minimum of 5 minutes is required in the performing of it. 2. Each thumb push has to be accompanied with an exhalation, breath-wise.

1. Sitting or standing, apply simultaneous medial thumb pressure from the sides of your body inwards into and at, the loins (soft area between lowest rib and upper rim of pelvis).
2. Apply as much pressure as you can endure, even if you create pain on both sides of the spine you are depressing, it is good – pain/discomfort can be worked-out.
3. You may move around a little with your thumbs – you are forcing blood, fluids, oxygen, the life force, and any other substance yet to be discovered, into the many structures of this area of rich resource.
4. As you apply pressure from outside in, with your thumbs or even index and middle fingers, you are exhaling at normal breathing speed. So accompany this thumb push movement with an exhalation each time, if not, the results of lining-up the pelvis will not be complete.
5. You need to perform this technique for at least 5 minutes for it to work well – no maximum time limit.
6. Execute this technique at least once a day – no maximum ceiling.
7. Do not labour your breathing; your breath should be easy and unforced, just as you breathe normally.

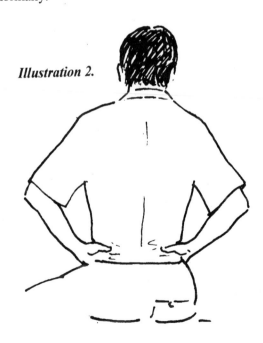

Illustration 2.

BACKCHAMP® (PELVIC CORRECTOR)

The function and purpose of: THE BACKCHAMP® is based on the premise that without pelvic stabilisation, even when segments of the spine are re-aligned, back-pain and other musculo-skeletal aches and pains will continue always.

The spine must sit on a base [pelvis] that is horizontal, to enable it [the spine] to remain vertical. The pelvis becomes dysfunctional, and tilts, amongst other things, to one side. This dysfunction is commonplace. What is engendered is an oblique angled pelvis, and now the segments of the spine, sitting on this oblique angled pelvis, have to twist and turn to compensate for pelvic distortion. In addition leg length discrepancy occurs.

It is this distortion that helps to create all the misery of musculo-skeletal disorders such as with lumbago, sciatica, frozen shoulder, knee and neck pain and more....

The good news is that it is possible for most of us to maintain our pelvises ourselves with a simple technique. This technique is called: 'The Regulator'. THE BACKCHAMP® assists with ease and comfort in executing this 'Regulator' technique safely.

THE 'REGULATOR' TECHNIQUE WORKS WITH THE BACKCHAMP® THUS: Lying down or sitting, with feet together acting as a fulcrum and the knees placed such as to be against the outside of the flaps of the BACKCHAMP®, the knees are brought together with great force against these flaps which counteract them. In this way the sacro-iliac joints give way fractionally as does the joint at the pubic bone. What happens now is that the specialised ligaments involved in the stabilisation of the pelvis, re-set themselves, as they have previously been distorted and have contributed to the cause of the dysfunctional pelvis at the outset. The re-setting of the ligaments happens immediately, and the whole pelvis re-aligns itself. This is all performed in Part A. You are able to rotate the Backchamp® device for comfort against the flesh and bone of the knees both in this Part A, and also Part B:-

In Part B, the knees are brought together and placed against the inner sides of the flaps, and forced outwards against them. Thus, the pelvis is made to return its own joints to perfection. The pelvis is now vertical where it should be, and horizontal where it should be. Therefore, it is aligned, and freedom from pain is enjoyed. However, the process above has to be repeated several times a day for a year or more, as the body must eventually change its habit of derangement cultivated over years by bony distortion. The reasons for these distortions are too great to include in this advice sheet, but access to some reasons why can be viewed in my manual: Correct Your Pelvis and Heal Your Back-pain.

ADDITIONAL BENEFITS when applying BACKCHAMP®

- Strengthens adductor and abductor muscles in thighs

- Helps to equalise strength in both legs

- Strengthens pelvic floor muscles

POTENTIAL CONTRA-INDICATIONS

- With pregnancy, it is very possible to continue or begin 'Pelvic Correction', only to be sensible with its application. The infant inside your abdomen will enjoy a womb that is angularly both horizontal and vertical, and not oblique as is the usual case, engendering potential disorders during the full term of the infant.

- Whether one or both hips have been replaced, again, requires some common sense as when applying the 'Pelvic Correction' Technique. The push and pull may have to be not as great as indicated overleaf.

DISCLAIMER

The BACKCHAMP® when applied properly should re-align the pelvis and therefore help to eliminate pain or at least reduce it. Harm cannot manifest using the machine as its action goes with and not against the body's natural proclivities. Even so, it is advised to obtain other expert advice, as from a medical doctor, before attempting the implementation of the 'Regulator Technique' indicated. The patentee and the manufacturer hereby disclaim liability for loss or injury sustained by an individual when applying the technique described, with the use of the BACKCHAMP®.

SOME REASONS WHY WE SUFFER PELVIC INSTABILITY

**By now, readers of this manual will be
pondering the question: "why is my pelvis unstable". The following teachings
should help them to understand <u>some</u> of the reasons why:**

*Most of you have your pelvis 'out-of-kilter' and consequent musculo-skeletal
pain. The reasons why, are, that all kinds of life stresses take their toll. Actually,
any reason the reader may hit upon will be the right one. There are a plethora of
reasons: from the habit of approaching a stairway always with the same leg, to
sitting on a sofa with the back not being upright.*

Oriental medicine theory states that **kidney** *Chi* rules, amongst other things, the
bones and the joints. Whatever affects the kidneys and depletes them energetically
will partly have its consequence in the tissue that the kidneys rule, namely: bones
and joints. The first bones to sublux/distort when kidney *Chi* is deficient would be
the components of the weight-bearing sacro-iliac joints. Namely: the ilium, sacrum
and L5*. The Kidneys are adversely affected by: illness; fear; lack of security,
financial and otherwise; shock; overwork; and the illusion most of us are under and
that is: the thought that: <u>'there isn't enough, and always a dearth of resources'</u> ♦.

Spleen *Chi,* rules, amongst other things, the muscles and muscle systems. When
spleen *Chi* is deficient, several muscles, usually the most overworked, will become
either too flaccid and/or tend to spasm/shorten. Because of this, the components of
joints, as mentioned above, may be pulled out-of-place by tight, and even loose
muscles, and especially by a dysfunctional **Psoas** and **Piriformis** muscle. The most
common joint components becoming displaced/subluxed are the sacro-iliac joints
and, the joint of the lumbo-sacral junction* (there are others displacements within
the spine however). The spleen is adversely affected by: worry; anxiety; over-caring;
anguish; overwork and the most common and destructive thought that: <u>'the worst
will always happen'</u> ♦.

Liver *Chi,* rules, amongst other things, the tendons and ligaments. When liver *Chi*
is out-of-balance the tendons and ligaments will not be nourished fully, and as a
result, tend to become too dry, fibrous and inflexible. This will have the affect of
shortening or over stretching particular ligaments and tendons, and this may lead to
subluxed/distorted joints also; commonly at the sacro-iliac joints and, at the lumbo-
sacral junction. The Liver is adversely affected by: anger; frustration; 'being put-
upon' and the mistaken notion many of us have: <u>'that life is burdensome and fraught
with rigour'</u> ♦.

Subluxation inevitably engenders misalignment of the pelvis

*The Heart, Lungs and Colon will also be involved in their respective ways; any book on Chinese Medicine will give
the various clues to this. However, I recommend reading: The Foundations of Chinese Medicine by Giovanni Maciocia
♦Recommended reading books: Conversations With God by Neal Donald Walsch, Various books by:
Deepak Chopra... * View Illustrations. 3 & 5a.*

Chapter Two

> *It is necessary to understand the real purpose of this manual. And that is to bring to the attention of both the layman and the professional that it is more than possible to move gently ones own bones/joints and especially the pelvic joints into their correct position without pain or trauma, and without the thrusting or the percussive methods employed with some therapies. Even so, osseous adjustments will contribute to pelvic stability following Pelvic Correction.*
> *Why re-align the pelvis? Because 9 out of every 10 cases of back-pain and additional musculo-skeletal problems are due to pelvic instability/slippage.*

In Chapter One, you have learned how to control your pelvis, or at least reduced your aches and pains by diligently following the details of the first techniques given that teach you particular practices. You may now take your knowledge further if you so wish, or simply glean additional understanding of the subject in question.

Re-establishing the pelvis' integrity is generally not the problem. The difficulty is that the pelvis does not stay in its true position even following Pelvic Correction, assuming the therapist has made the correction! It requires **self-help** work to gain the stability required.

In addition, even in the acute pain stage of your back having just 'given way', and having caused you to flounder and suffer the indignity of being unable to move, you may still perform and/or get help from a friend or partner to assist you to perform, the special techniques outlined in this unique manual to re-align the pelvis. Thereby, helping you to recover much more quickly than it would be as in the normal circumstance.

You cannot do harm with these gentle techniques. If after performing them, and you are much relieved and after a few days or weeks things go terribly wrong pain-wise, it is not because of the use of these techniques. **It is for the following reasons:**

1. You need to try harder and more frequently the operation of the techniques. Do not be afraid of this because the techniques applied need to 'break through' muscular contraction to re-align the pelvis again. Try a one-off very powerful 'Regulator' to 'break through'. Always re-assess. See Chapter 4.

2. You should follow-up by having the whole spine re-aligned by an Osteopath or Chiropractor - but you are the one who can deal with the pelvis, and the total results will be excellent for you health-wise, and in pain reduction.

3. Following this, if there is still discomfort even when the pelvis is aligned, you should consult your physician to have your spine x-rayed should there be an additional pathological reason for your back-pain.

4. You will probably need a thorough body workout. Receiving deep shiatsu therapy, or any like bodywork will help release tight muscles and tendons that are involved in the cause your aches and pains in the first place.

> *The following texts describe the <u>real</u> situation with regard to pelvic distortion being responsible for 9 out of every 10 cases of musculo-skeletal pain, i.e. lower, middle, upper back; pain on either side of spine usually at waist level; lumbago; sciatic pain side and back, and side of thigh; including other curious aches and pains in other bodily places:*

Other than the unfortunate experience of injury (contusion) to a part of the musculo-skeletal system and/or simple muscle sprain, almost without exception the distortion of the pelvis is responsible for your musculo-skeletal aches and pains: being **the foundation of the skeletal frame**, it is essential that the pelvis remains neatly horizontal in its true position. This enables the segments (vertebrae) of the spine to sit square-on above it [pelvis]. **Thus, a healthy flexible spine is enjoyed, because the spine and the sacrum/coccyx are exactly <u>vertical</u> and in-line, by virtue of a <u>horizontal</u> pelvic body, upon which they sit. View Page 13 (Healthy Upright Body)**.

Deep discomfort is experienced when the wings (ilia) of the pelvis move 'out of kilter' because of instability of the sacral and lumbar components, and adjacent specialised ligaments, including certain adjoining muscles. These dysfunctions are actually very commonplace. **(Read page 9 and View Illustrations 3 & 5 a/b)**

However, the problem is a serious one as well as being universal amongst the different populations of the world. The consequences of a misaligned pelvis, the spinal column now sitting above and on a distorted base [the pelvis], are to create misery, discomfort and pain; as well as interference with an active life to the point of limiting the enjoyment of it, often quite suddenly and unexpectedly.

In addition, because the spinal segments must also bend and turn to accommodate this dysfunctional base [the pelvis/sacrum], various spinal nerves definitely will be constricted/snagged and therefore their electrical and biological impulses severely reduced as they exit/enter from particular areas of that spine. Also, those <u>structures</u> which these <u>restricted</u> nerves supply, will in turn produce pain and limited movement; namely with your:

Shoulder area; upper arms; elbows; wrists; neck; cranial base (skull), and more.

<u>Inevitably, adverse visceral affects have to be taken into consideration also when nerve supply is restricted.</u>

"Aunt Agatha's demeanour now was rather like that of one who, picking daisies at the railway, has just caught the down express in the small of the back".

The Inimitable Jeeves (1923) (By permission of A.P.Watt Ltd., on behalf of the Trustees of the Wodehouse Estate)

SKELETAL DISTORTIONS
DUE TO A RIGHT SIDE "DROPPED" PELVIS

FRONT VIEW

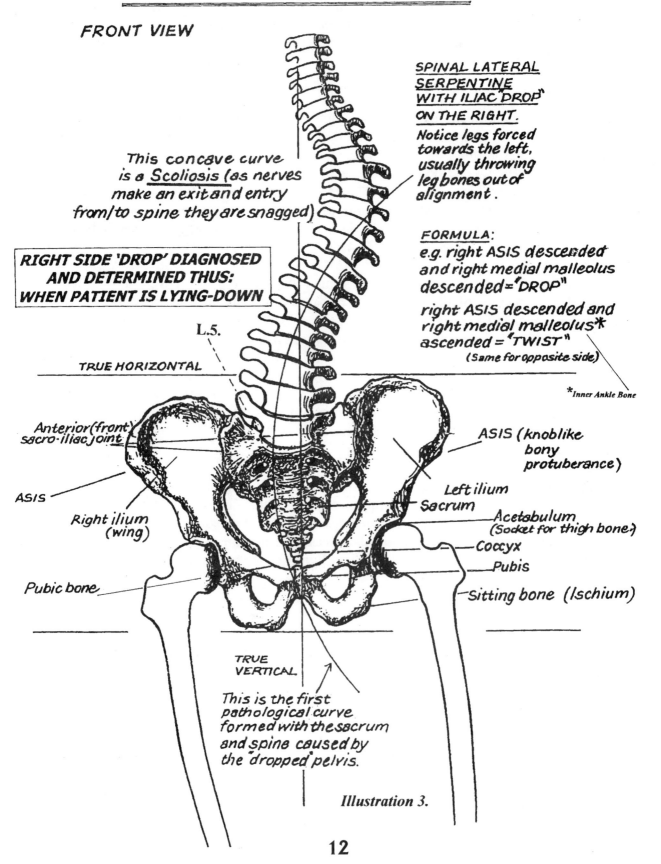

SPINAL LATERAL SERPENTINE WITH ILIAC "DROP" ON THE RIGHT.
Notice legs forced towards the left, usually throwing leg bones out of alignment.

This concave curve is a <u>Scoliosis</u> (as nerves make an exit and entry from/to spine they are snagged)

FORMULA:
e.g. right ASIS descended and right medial malleolus descended = "DROP"

right ASIS descended and right medial malleolus* ascended = "TWIST"
(Same for opposite side)

RIGHT SIDE 'DROP' DIAGNOSED AND DETERMINED THUS: WHEN PATIENT IS LYING-DOWN

*Inner Ankle Bone

L.5.

TRUE HORIZONTAL

Anterior (front) sacro-iliac joint

ASIS (knoblike bony protuberance)

ASIS

Left ilium

Sacrum

Right ilium (wing)

Acetabulum (Socket for thigh bone)

Coccyx

Pubis

Pubic bone

Sitting bone (Ischium)

TRUE VERTICAL

This is the first pathological curve formed with the sacrum and spine caused by the 'dropped' pelvis.

Illustration 3.

12

A COMPREHENSIBLE ILLUSTRATION OF HOW A HUMAN SPINE SUBLUXES (THE BODY IS FACING THE READER)

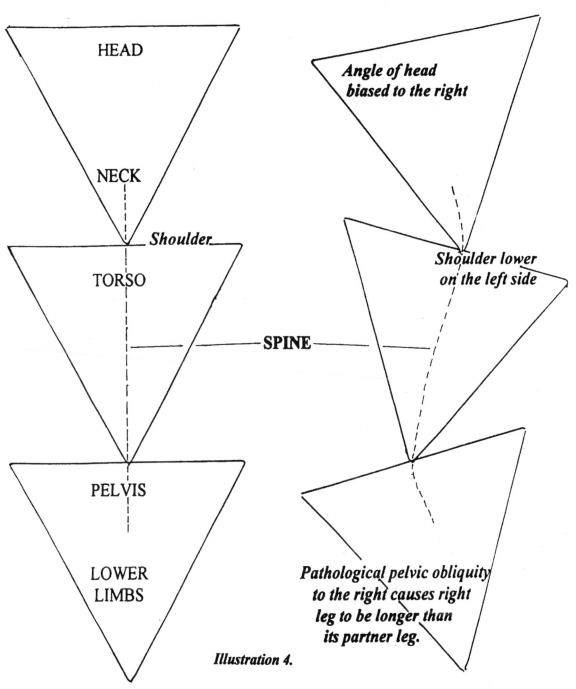

HEALTHY UP-RIGHT BODY

PELVIC 'DROP' RIGHT-SIDE

CAUSES ANGULAR DISRUPTION AND SCOLIOTIC SPINE

HEAD

NECK

Angle of head biased to the right

Shoulder

TORSO

Shoulder lower on the left side

SPINE

PELVIS

LOWER LIMBS

Pathological pelvic obliquity to the right causes right leg to be longer than its partner leg.

Illustration 4.

13

SPINE VERSUS PELVIS

Philosophically, osteopathy and to some extent chiropractic consider the <u>condition</u> of the spine itself to be the <u>determinant</u> of an aligned or a misaligned pelvis.

There is much credence to this idea. After all, in 50% of cases, a trained therapist may correct your pelvis by re–aligning your spine alone - not having to touch your pelvis at all.

However, the pelvis has its own life and intelligence, and this becomes apparent when you work with it, and, as the foundation of the skeletal frame, will dislocate for umpteen reasons: your spine or parts of your spine will suffer as a result. Even so, you yourself are able to correct your pelvis thereby helping to maintain reasonably an aligned spine and therefore its health as well.

The pelvis is the one item you are able to adjust yourself, whilst for most of us it is equally not possible to do so in the same way with our own spines, owing to the natural position and placing of our bones.

It is true that for many reasons, such as with diet, and especially a diet very high in acid content (as opposed to alkaline content. Read APPENDICES pages 59/63), a given spine begins to deteriorate over time and thereby causes back-pain, that may have little to do with a pelvis distorted or straight. Even so, in the majority of cases the distorted pelvis will have repercussions affecting the spine adversely, such as to engender the many types of pathologies that plague it.

"You know you are getting old
when your pelvis goes-out
more often than you do"

The arguments from Page 10 onwards, reveal the problems 'above the belt'. The problems 'below the belt' are also debilitating: if you have ever wondered why your knee does not heal and why you have twisted your ankle many times, and why your foot hurts; then you will understand that your leg bones are out-of- alignment, as dictated by your distorted pelvis. In other words, until your pelvis is re-aligned your knee, ankle and foot will never really heal properly. How can they, when the joints belonging to these three areas of the leg are forced not to align.

Most of you who read this (80% approximately) should be able to perform the following Pelvic Correction Techniques successfully provided you carry-out diligently the exact instructions outlined.

However, note the importance of the following three points:

First: For the purpose of simplification, I am dealing with only **two main types of pelvic dysfunction** that give rise to back-pain. There are some variations on these two main types and, these variations are understood and dealt with by professionals, and others trained in the author's Pelvic Correction Techniques. Otherwise, as stated, for most of us, it is possible to correct the pelvis ourselves understanding these **two main dysfunctions.**

Second: 60% of your aches and pains can be eliminated almost immediately or at least within a few days following Pelvic Correction. A high quality of energy will be released interiorly which will help you to feel good again, and, curiously, conditions such as with headache and digestive problems can clear-up completely or at least be ameliorated. This is because the skeletal frame when assisted back to its pristine straightness, helps the nerve impulses to be more regulated. Thus, all body structures are supplied uniformly with these healthy impulses without the usual constrictions engendered by misaligned bones.

(And for those who understand energy from the oriental point of view: "Chi" is now flowing smoothly as it should)

Third: Correcting the pelvic girdle is relatively easy. The difficulty here for most of us, is that it [the pelvis] will not stay in its true position following correction. Therefore, persistent, diligent daily homework possibly for a year or two or three, is necessary to obtain the stability of the pelvis as desired. Hence: freedom from back-pain and more.

Chapter Three

TYPES OF PELVIC DYSFUNCTIONS

> ***Below, are explanations of the two main types of pelvic dysfunctions/lesions* which represent an important part of the essence of this manual:***

A 'drop' lesion – a pelvic inferior osseous prolapsus
A 'twist' lesion – a pelvic anterior osseous 'torsion'

A **'drop'** lesion happens when one wing (ilium) of the pelvis has **'dropped'** towards the ground (inferior), **driven by unstable ligaments, sacrum and lumbar segments**, and has taken the leg with it, because of course it is attached to the pelvis via the upper part of the thigh bone (femur). If this 'drop' is say ¼ inch in measurement, then the leg, on the same side will have dropped ¼ inch as well, and therefore it will be ¼ inch longer than its partner leg.

The consequences of this are not good below or above the 'belt' because the whole spine is now sitting on an oblique base (pelvis) and not one that is healthy and <u>horizontal</u>. The effect is one of a side-to-side serpentine shape forced onto the spine. (View Illustrations 3 & 4)

A **'twist'** lesion is engendered when a wing of the pelvis has *'torsioned'* **forwards**, again, **driven by unstable ligaments, sacrum and lumbar segments**, so that its upper part has inordinately moved frontwards and its lower part has swung backwards, lifting the leg headwards in the process, because it is [the leg] attached of course. If the torsion discrepancy is say ¼ inch then the leg will have been **shortened/lifted** by that ¼ inch in relation to its partner leg. (View Illustrations 5a & 5b) Note: the opposite ilium would also have *'torsioned'* **backwards**.

Again, the consequences are very unfavourable, below and above the 'belt'. Not only is the spine now sitting on an oblique base as for the 'drop' and therefore suffers a side-to-side bend, but also that base (sacrum) is now forced to twist slightly around a vertical axis causing the spine to **exaggerate** its normal backwards and frontwards **'S'** bend to a much greater degree pathologically. The total effect on the spine therefore, is one of a corkscrew form, and the creation of a lordosis and scoliosis is inevitable!

> ***lesion, subluxation, and dysfunction** are used interchangeably; all having a
> similar meaning which is: dysfunction.

> **This is an additional reminder as to the necessity of adhering to the exact instructions outlined for each technique. In this way, you will not only execute a given technique properly, but you will also understand the reasons for its creation. Importantly, you should become pain-free when you apply precision to your work.**

When a given pelvis suffers the 'twist' (torsion) of both ilia (wings), it is possible only to illustrate this dysfunction by looking downwards at the pelvis from above. That is, from a superior position:

Lines of viewing

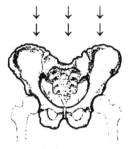

The following front (anterior) view illustration 5a, represents the healthy normal pelvis when actually viewed from above [superiorly]:

THE BROKEN LINES REPRESENT THE HEALTHY COMPONENTS OF THE PELVIS AT THEIR TRUE ANGLES

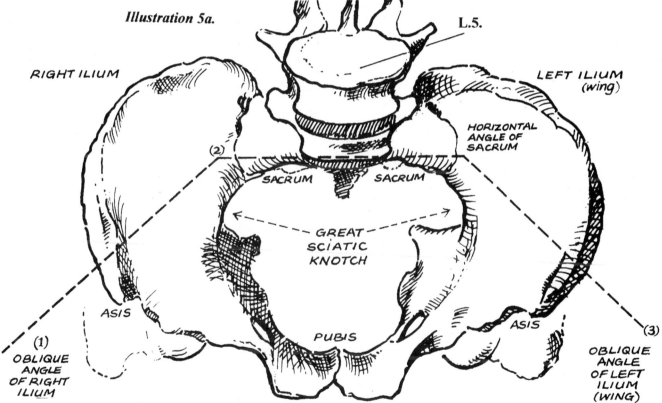

On the opposite page Illust. 5 b, the 3 broken lines, again, represent each major pelvic component, but pathologically placed (dysfunctional), as they are when the pelvis suffers a right-side 'twist'(torsion). That is, the right ilium (wing) has twisted forward anteriorly.

The sacro-iliac joints tend to be over-flexible, allowing this dysfunction (distortion) to happen.

*If a left-side 'twist' occurs (left ilium twisted forwards anteriorly) all factors indicated are in reverse.

17

The broken lines (1), (2), and (3) in Illust. 5b, represent the pathological (dysfunctional) angles the 3 major pelvic components suffer (right ilium, sacrum, left ilium) when a right-sided 'twist' occurs.

Note: *These pathological angles all occur <u>in one movement</u>, which includes the superior or up-lifting of the right side of the pelvis, and this accounts for the shortening of the right leg, compared to the left leg, by virtue of that leg being lifted by the pelvis on that side. All in reverse if a left-side 'twist' occurs.*

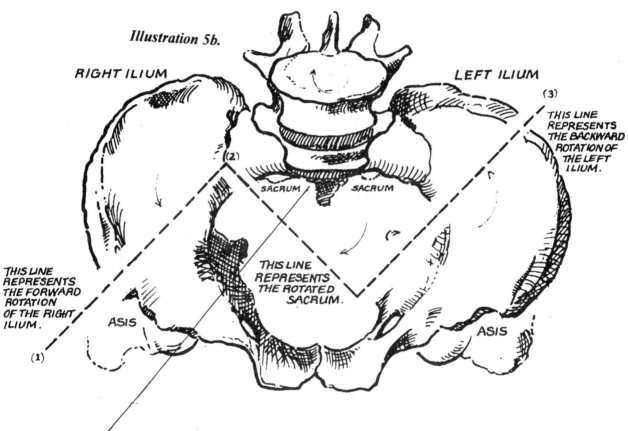

Illustration 5b.

RIGHT ILIUM

LEFT ILIUM

(3)

THIS LINE REPRESENTS THE BACKWARD ROTATION OF THE LEFT ILIUM.

(2)

SACRUM

SACRUM

THIS LINE REPRESENTS THE FORWARD ROTATION OF THE RIGHT ILIUM.

THIS LINE REPRESENTS THE ROTATED SACRUM.

ASIS

ASIS

(1)

This sacrum will swing around on its vertical axis as per broken middle line (2). The left ilium rotates on its horizontal axis backwards posteriorly as per broken line (3) forming a deep hollow at the back, giving rise to a lordosis especially visible from left side of patient, note the V shape of the broken lines (2) and (3). The right ilium rotates forward anteriorly on its horizontal axis as per broken line (1) causing an upside-down V.

An unstable sacral component and lower lumbar segments (vertebrae) are part of the cause of the 'drop' and the 'twist' lesions. (See Kidneys Page 9   ).   A certain percentage of this pelvic instability is due to the tightness and/or looseness of pertinent muscles (See Spleen Page 9   ) such as with the *Gluteus Maximus; Piriformis; Psoas Major; Iliacus; Quadratus Lumborum.* Also, take into consideration the stiffness and/or weakness of relevant tendons, and ligaments that hold the various structures together.

* All in reverse if a left-sided 'twist'.

18

SIDE VIEW OF PELVIS

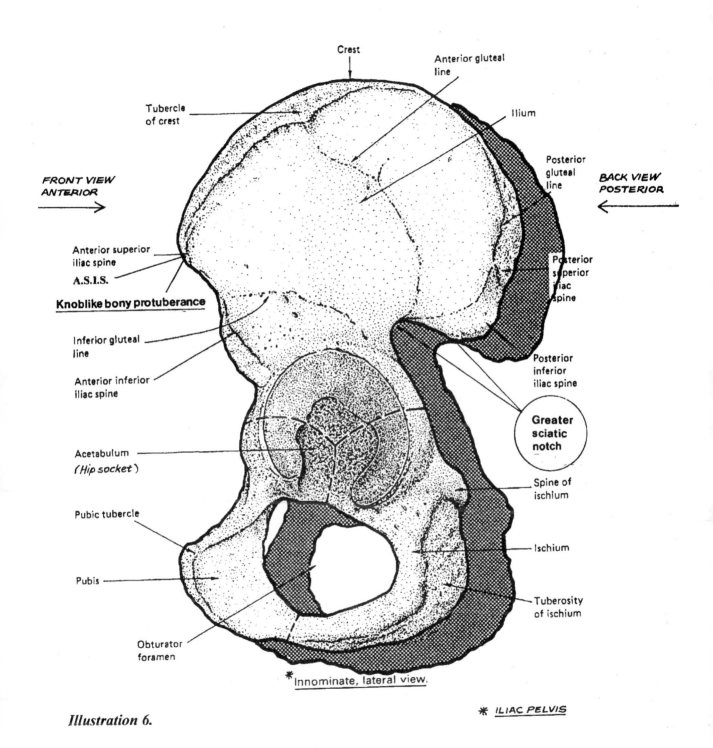

Crest

Anterior gluteal line

Tubercle of crest

Ilium

Posterior gluteal line

FRONT VIEW
ANTERIOR
→

BACK VIEW
POSTERIOR
←

Anterior superior iliac spine

A.S.I.S.

Knoblike bony protuberance

Posterior superior iliac spine

Inferior gluteal line

Anterior inferior iliac spine

Posterior inferior iliac spine

Greater sciatic notch

Acetabulum
(Hip socket)

Spine of ischium

Pubic tubercle

Ischium

Pubis

Tuberosity of ischium

Obturator foramen

❋ Innominate, lateral view.

❋ ILIAC PELVIS

Illustration 6.

19

Illustration 7.

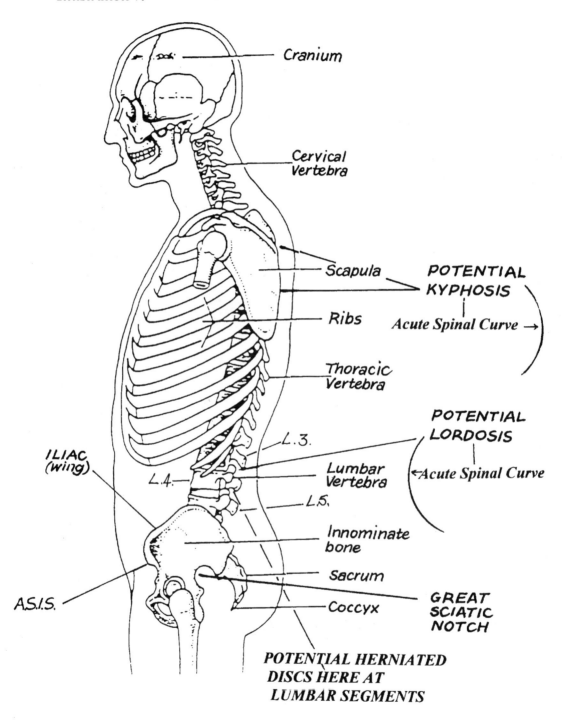

Cranium

Cervical
Vertebra

Scapula

POTENTIAL
KYPHOSIS

Acute Spinal Curve →

Ribs

Thoracic
Vertebra

POTENTIAL
LORDOSIS

L.3.

←Acute Spinal Curve

ILIAC
(wing)

Lumbar
Vertebra

L.4.

L.5.

Innominate
bone

Sacrum

GREAT
SCIATIC
NOTCH

A.S.I.S.

Coccyx

**POTENTIAL HERNIATED
DISCS HERE AT
LUMBAR SEGMENTS**

Chapter Four

It is possible for 80% of the population of the world to diagnose what type of pelvic lesion they suffer, and to practise the solution to this if they adhere to the following: (View Illustrations 8, 9, & 10)

SELF-ASSESSMENT AS TO LEG LENGTH DIFFERENCE AND NAMING THE DYSFUNCTION INVOLVED:

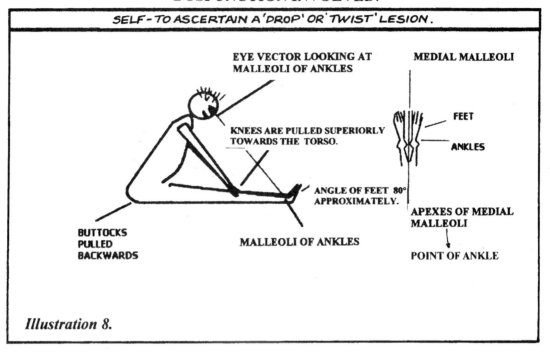

Illustration 8.

1. With legs together directly out in front of torso, and in line with the torso, i.e. neither to the left nor to the right, lean the whole torso forwards towards the feet, keeping the back as straight as is possible. (Similar to the Hatha-Yoga posture forward bend: Paschimottanasana).

2. Legs should be as straight as possible by pulling-up knees, i.e. knee-caps pulled towards your torso. This will help keep legs unbent.

3. It is essential now to pull backwards both buttocks, one at a time, using your hands, i.e. right hand under right buttock pull muscle out backwards, and same with left hand under left buttock. This will help legs to fall flush with the ground or couch you are sitting on as well as enabling your torso to move further forward.

4. Look to malleoli (inner ankle bones). Are both apex points of malleoli (eminences) in-line? This requires a cold dispassionate look. Get someone to look for you, if this is difficult to do, or use a ruler.

5. Whichever leg is shorter indicates either a 'twist' affecting that very leg, or a 'drop' on the opposite leg. Applying the relevant techniques (chapter 5), by a process of elimination, pelvic correction will be obtained. Try the 'twist' technique, on the shorter leg, and if this does not work because pain has not gone when upright, try 'drop' technique on longer leg.

6. Of course the same formula applies if the other leg is shorter.

7. Running this same sequence again will confirm if both legs are now aligned.

8. If both legs are of equal length now, your pelvis is aligned, walk-about for a few minutes, and you should notice a favourable difference.

Note, that fractional differences matter. Even a 1mm. difference matters! Self-assess daily.

There is an alternative even quicker way of assessing leg-length discrepancy. It means sitting on your heels/haunches. You need only to do this briefly, ('Seiza' posture in the Japanese tradition, and 'Thunderbolt' posture in the Yoga Tradition). (See Illustrations 9 & 10)

1. Look at the tips of both knees you will see immediately which knee is extended further than its partner knee.
2. Use a ruler if unsure, your eye should show you any difference in extension.
3. As above, the shorter knee means a 'twist' on that side or a 'drop' on the extended knee on the other side.
4. As above, by a process of elimination try first the 'twist' technique rectification on the shorter side, and if this does not work:
5. Try the 'drop' technique rectification on (chapter 5) the extended side.

Note again, a fractional difference matters! Self-assess daily.
See an Osteopath or Chiropractor if uncertain. Make the corrections yourself, following treatments.

You may also assess, in the same way, for simplicity, sitting on a straight chair. Sit upright and square-on at the edge of the chair, feet together exactly, and check knee differences, use a ruler for accuracy to elicit any disparity.

Illustration number 8 is probably the most accurate out of the three, assessment-wise. Do not be surprised to find that the dislocation of the pelvis to be on the opposite side of where your pain is, this is not unusual.

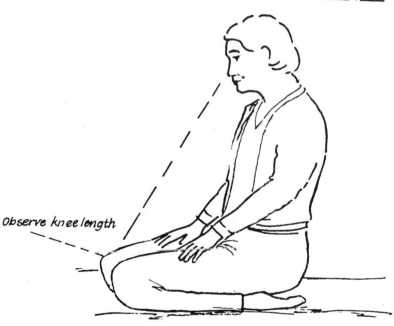

Self-assessment Technique

Observe knee length

Note: Left is shorter than right!

Illustration 9

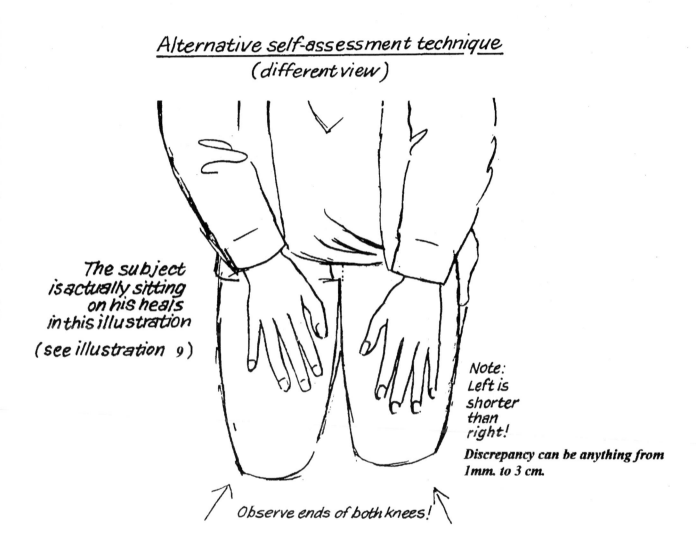

Alternative self-assessment technique
(different view)

The subject is actually sitting on his heals in this illustration

(see illustration 9)

Note:
Left is shorter than right!

Discrepancy can be anything from 1mm. to 3 cm.

Observe ends of both knees!

Illustration 10

TO SUMMARISE THE CONTENTS OF CHAPTER FOUR:

- There are three good techniques for self-assessing leg length discrepancy, which may lead to your knowing the type of pelvic dislocation you suffer.
- The first illustration #8 page 21 - the forward bend, is actually the best, but may be the most difficult to perform.
- The following technique, sitting on your heals, may be easier to perform for some of you. And it works very well.
- The last technique is the easiest to execute, though it may not be the most accurate. You have to keep both thighs still, once you are sitting on the edge of the chair.
- Not all these techniques agree with one another, it all depends on whether your sitting bones are equal in height, morphically (physical form) speaking. If two of the techniques agree in a diagnosis, that conclusion is the one to go for.

Several readers will be wondering how they may diagnose other people's pelvic misalignment. Absolute diagnosis as to whether a 'twist' or a 'drop' is involved, may only be ascertained when a person is face-upwards (supine). The reason for this is too convoluted to explain in this manual. There are, four reference points employed in diagnosis in this way, and they are: the two A.S.I.S. points, and the two medial malleoli points (inner ankle bones). View illustrations 3,6, & 8.

In truth, diagnosis in this way can only be taught in a workshop/Course situation, as there is a need for much practice under supervision with the use of these points in diagnosis. Therefore, only self-assessment can be given in this manual.

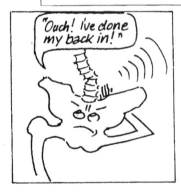

"Ouch! I've done my back in!"

Patrick the Pelvis...

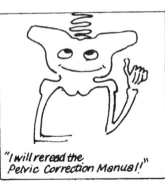

"I will reread the Pelvic Correction Manual!"

"Great! I can walk straight from now on!"

Chapter Five

THE RECTIFICATION TECHNIQUES FOR PELVIC CORRECTION

When you apply the technique for the '**drop**' (if you suffer a 'drop') you do the following: (Illustration 11. #1)

- The apparent longer leg should be brought towards you flexed (bent) so that the **bent knee** itself is facing the ceiling 85 to 90° but again towards you not away from you.

- With one hand over the other, as per sketch #1, Illustration.11 place hands against the upright thigh near the knee.

- Take an in-breath, and hold this breath for a count of 14 (medium speed 2 counts per second) and from the first count of **1,** you begin to push the upright thigh away from you using hands to do so, but do not let the thigh move away from you. Thus, you create a push/pull counterforce during the count of 14. It appears that nothing is happening because the counterforce is stopping the thigh from moving, as it should. What is happening though, is that the pelvis is being lifted fractionally in the direction towards your head and therefore pelvic correction is now being performed. Some real force is required!

- Repeat this whole process 4 more times. Diligent practice will produce the desired results. Make it as a military operation then it will work splendidly for you.

- Keep the head down/resting throughout.

For those interested in the mechanics of this: the deep 'psoas' muscle on that side is engaged, and thus it lifts superiorly that side of the pelvis to which it is attached.

Explanation:

The reason the breath is held and then released for each of the 5 turns is because the push/pull exercise requires some strength to execute, and holding the breath enables you to achieve this.

The reason why you count to 14 with each turn is that with each turn you give sufficient time, fractionally, bit by bit for the pelvis to be lifted superiorly in the direction towards your head, which is exactly what is needed, very desperately so.

Remember that the whole pelvis has literally dropped on one side in the direction towards the feet and has extended the leg on that side abnormally.

You may wish to add another technique for the 'drop': (see illustration 11 #2). This is always to be performed only on the other leg, in other words on the side that does not have the problem.

- With an exhalation, stretch the arm and the shorter leg (same side) in opposite directions hold this stretch for three breaths after which release on exhalation.

- **In illustration 11 (#2) the 'drop' is on the left side.**

- Note that the leg should be pushed away from you; pushing out from the heel.

- The arm on that side should be above your head, and pushing in opposite direction from the leg on that side. Repeat four more times.

- This technique **must only** be performed on the unaffected opposite leg to the 'drop' or you will cause an additional pelvic problem. This particular technique **is** an exception, but works well.

When you apply the technique for the 'twist', (if you suffer a 'twist') do the following: (See illustration 11 #3 'twist')

- With the apparent shorter leg, bring it flexed (bent) at the knee tightly towards you so that this leg's knee is as near to the armpit as is possible, that is, a little away from the body. You do this by wrapping the <u>crook of the elbow</u> over and around the shin (slightly below the knee) and pull tightly towards the armpit with the help of the other arm. Hold tight for **two minutes**. The pelvis should correct itself. Great strength should be applied pulling your bent leg towards you.

- You are lying down, face-up (supine), keep your head resting throughout.

For those who wish to know what is happening here: the femur (thigh bone) is being used as a lever to rotate back and backwards the ilium that has 'torsioned' forwards pathologically.

N.B. Book: Soft Tissue Manipulation by Leon Chaitow (Muscle Energy Techniques)

Illustration 11

DROP

1.

Flexed leg even better if
more towards your chest

You may alternatively push this thigh
away from you, pushing from mid-
thigh, if this is more comfortable.

Push/pull equally. Hold the
in-breath counting to 14 then
relax the breath and also the
push/pull. Immediately begin
the process again. Total 6 times

2.

The limbs on this side are pushed in
opposite directions, and held thus for
three breaths. Push leg away from HEEL

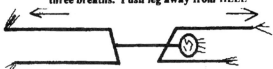

Do not perform on the problem side, only
the opposite side to it. See notes

TWIST

3.

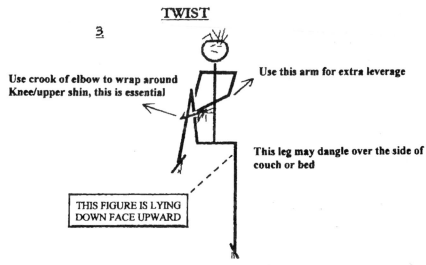

Use crook of elbow to wrap around
Knee/upper shin, this is essential

Use this arm for extra leverage

This leg may dangle over the side of
couch or bed

THIS FIGURE IS LYING
DOWN FACE UPWARD

Pull tightly towards armpit for 2 mins.
When this technique begins to feel easier
to perform, it may not work so well, in
which case pull an additional 10% or more
towards your armpit

Notes to the 'twist' technique:

- Breathe at normal breathing speed throughout the two-minute hold. (This technique is very different from the others given).

- Within say, 4 days, if it feels easier to perform, it may not work so well. It means you have to pull your flexed leg more powerfully towards you, an additional 10%, in fact, and possibly slightly further away from the torso. You should be pulling **very hard** anyway.

- You may add the following to work simultaneously with the above: the leg that is longer, the leg that is actually not involved should be allowed to hang downwards loosely towards the floor. This can only be performed therefore on a bed or a couch. Adding this may make a difference in the success of the result of this technique.

- There should always be a feeling of strain when executing this one.

Some of you will find this 'twist' Correction Technique difficult to do. If so, try the following way:

1. When applying the technique above you are supine in position (face-up). Now rotate 180° to prone position (face-down), and in identical posture as above, but without the arms wrapped around flexed leg.

2. It now looks as though you are bowing to Mecca, except that the leg not involved, is straight-out behind you.

3. Your flexed thigh, on the side that suffers the 'twist', is almost underneath your torso, however, it could also be a little away from the torso, a little away to the side.

4. In this way, the natural weight of the torso brings you closer towards the floor/ground and your own flexed thigh. Thus, your work is done for you, by virtue of your torso's weight.

5. Again, the correction will take one and a half to two minutes holding this posture. Keep the forehead on the floor if possible, and arms out in front of you.

TO SUMMARISE THE CONTENTS OF CHAPTER FIVE:

- There are several Pelvic Correction techniques that help bring the pelvis back to its pristine position/condition.
- When dealing with a **'drop'** dislocation, which has been diagnosed by you, you have a choice of two correction techniques. Depending on your mood on a particular day, you may indeed choose the technique most suited to you on that day. There are more 'drop' techniques available, but these can only be taught in a workshop situation.
- You may perform the push/pull technique for the 'drop' sitting down, and this enables you to execute it on a plane, train, car, or in the office. It will act provisionally.
- Of course, when you are lying horizontally, this technique will work better.

- There are two techniques for the **'twist'** dislocation.
- There are more, but these may only be taught in a workshop situation.
- The first technique is not easy to execute for many of you, and there must be always a sense of strain with this one, to work efficiently. This means pulling the thigh tightly towards your torso/armpit.
- **You are lying down (supine) face-up for the above technique**.
- The alternative is easier and takes about two minutes to succeed also. Simply think in terms of an 180° about turn (prone, face downwards) and then proceed to do it. The flexed leg is now beneath your torso, though slightly away from the body [in some cases it would work directly underneath the torso]. The other leg not involved is straight out behind you, and just breath normally. Your own body weight does the business!

In addition to the 'Regulator' Technique as illustrated on page 6 at the beginning of this manual, you may choose two additional techniques, both of which may return the pelvis to its normal position whether it [pelvis] suffers a 'twist' or a 'drop':

Alexalign Technique may be performed in the same way as you perform the 'Regulator'. However, it requires some strength to push the feet against each other, and it really needs to be executed lying down. Even so, it is effective. Illustration 12.

Glencroft Technique may be performed in the same way as you perform the 'Regulator'. Again, this technique may only be performed lying down, and you have to assess which leg **appears** longer than its partner leg. Illustration 13.

A 'twist' and a 'drop' lesion cannot really occur together. That is, a mixture of both. You may suffer a 'drop' on Monday and a 'twist' on Tuesday. And this is how it goes 'so to speak'.

ALEXALIGN TECHNIQUE

This is an additional technique devised to return the pelvis to its proper balanced state whether you suffer a 'drop' or a 'twist' to the pelvis

This technique may only be executed lying down face-up (supine):

- As per illustration 1, below, bring feet together – knees pointing outwards
- Take a breath, hold this breath pushing both feet together against each other, counting up to 14 or 16
- Repeat this 4 times

As per illustration 2, second part, lock feet together, and:

- Try to pull legs apart, holding your in-breath for a count of 14 or 16
- Of course as the legs are locked at the feet, the legs cannot pull apart and **this is the point** of this part of the technique
- Repeat 3 times

This technique works in the same principle way the 'regulator' operates, accept that the 'Alexalign' may only be performed lying down, but no gadgets are required at all for it to be executed.

It is possible to strain too much **when applying push** to the legs in the first part of this technique. You will need to draw **back from this, and** adjust your strength accordingly.

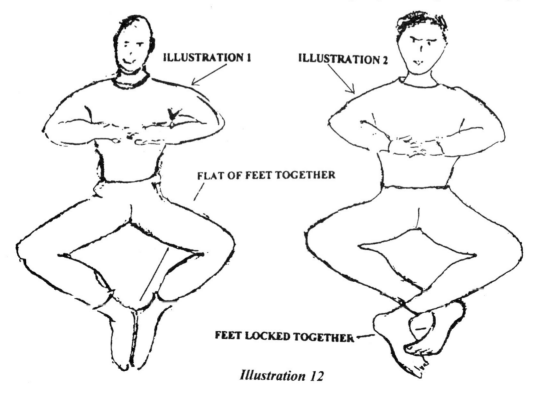

ILLUSTRATION 1   ILLUSTRATION 2

FLAT OF FEET TOGETHER

FEET LOCKED TOGETHER

Illustration 12

GLENCROFT TECHNIQUE FOR PELVIC CORRECTION

NOTE: IT IS AS WELL TO UNDERSTAND THAT ASSESSMENT OF LEG AND PELVIC DISCREPANCY MAY ONLY BE DIAGNOSED BY ANOTHER PERSON ACCURATELY WHEN THE PATIENT IS LYING-DOWN.

Lying down, and face upwards (supine), and you have assessed, say, a right 'drop' and perhaps you have had confirmation that you do have a right 'drop', so the right leg, therefore is **longer** than the left leg, place the left foot over the right foot, as per illustration below, and as you pull the right leg up superiorly from the hip, push down inferiorly the left leg from the hip, the left foot is pressing downwards now against the right foot and being restrained thus.

Try to keep both legs as straight as you can, and as with previous techniques explained. Breathe-in and hold your breath to a count of around the number 16 whilst pushing downwards with the left leg and pulling upwards with the right leg. Repeat at least 4 times using good strength. Your pelvis will rotate a bit and you may experience a click at your lower back.

Needless to say, if you suffer a left 'drop', and therefore your left leg is **longer** than your right leg, you would perform the reverse procedure by pushing downwards inferiorly the right leg and pulling-up superiorly the left leg with the right foot over the left foot.

Even with a 'twist', the **longer leg** is treated exactly as explained above, and the 'twist' problem is neutralized as with the 'drop'.

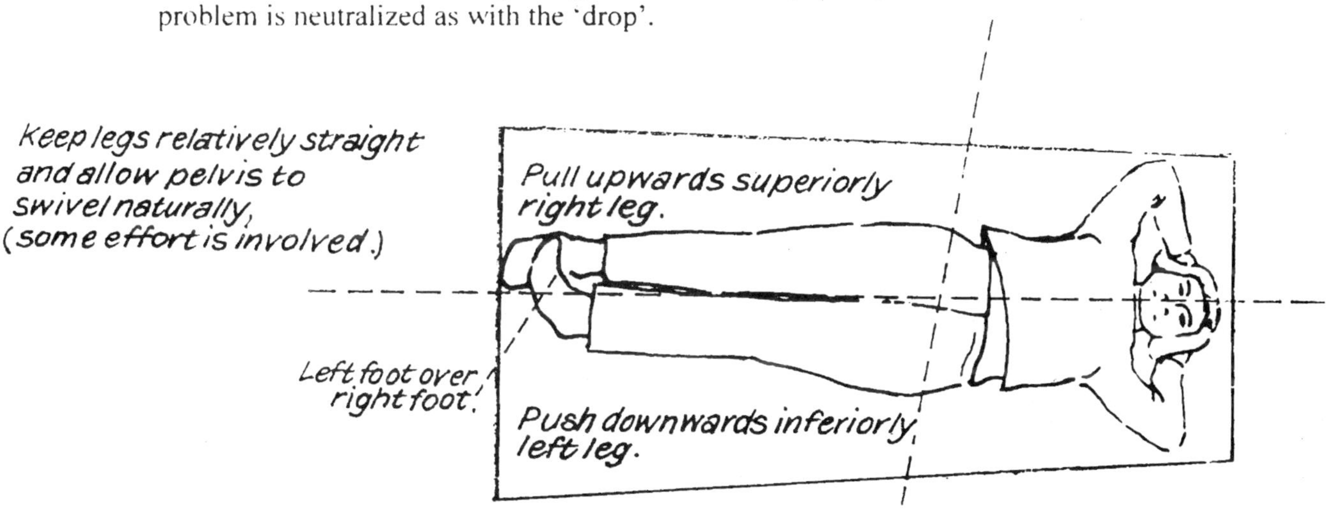

keep legs relatively straight and allow pelvis to swivel naturally, (some effort is involved.)

Pull upwards superiorly right leg.

Left foot over right foot!

Push downwards inferiorly left leg.

Illustration 13 **31**

Chapter Six

> *The techniques outlined in chapter five help <u>to return the pelvis position-wise</u>. The techniques below <u>assist stabilization of the pelvis</u> and just a few of these techniques will also return the pelvis to its proper aligned state. You may administer these techniques successfully yourself. They are proven and used by the author.*

STABILIZATION TECHNIQUES

- Lie on your side (recovery position) but on the side of the body not involved. This exposes the subluxed side you need to work with. Use a cushion for your head. (See Illustration 14 & 15)

- Now for a **fluid compression drive**: on this subluxed side, with **passive** hand placed at back, upper buttock, of sacro-iliac joint, apply the other **active** hand and especially that hand's fingers to point and to delve deep into the pelvic rim, that is, on the soft side of the bony knob-like part, known as the A.S.I.S.

- This is your landmark, but soft side only. Gently **dig** well into the ligaments/tendons/muscles deep inside that part of the abdomen. Always wear some clothing to protect your abdomen from your nails. Lying in this way allows you to dig deep into this particular area

- The hand at the back is also moving/pressing towards the digging hand, thus you have created a compressive type of movement (as though both hands are coming towards each other). **<u>Accompany this compressive movement and gentle but deep plunge with an exhalation at normal breathing speed. This is the speed at which you press inwards, in fact. Do not accelerate your breath.</u>**

- Altogether, you now have a rhythmic movement of both hands coming towards each other accompanied by an exhalation with that part of the pelvis in between both hands.

- You have an arc of about two and a half inches abdominally, within which to operate. You can work out any pain in this area back and front. You are stimulating the repair of tissue and especially the ligaments/muscles in this weakened place.

- Perform the above technique for 5 minutes at least. Both hands are **180°** **opposite** each other, this, is the correct vector between them.

FOLLOWING THE TECHNIQUE ABOVE:

- Now is the time, if you so wish, to execute the **fluid/energy drive technique**: point the active fingers to the sacro-iliac joint and using your mind envision/project energy (imagine electrical energy lines) from the active fingers through this joint to the passive hand/fingers of the other hand at the back.

- The hands and fingers may begin to pulse, and if they do, they will help to accelerate tissue repair. Even if they do not pulse, the healing process will still work - this operation only needs time to develop for you. You should begin to feel heat however. Which means you have made the connection.

- Perform for 5 minutes if possible. With this technique, both hands may be slightly off the body or just touching it. Both hands are 180° opposite each other. This is the correct vector between them. View Illustrations 14,15 & 16.

- Note that the best results seem to occur when the receiving hand's fingers are slightly apart from one another and that the active hand's fingers are projecting energy towards these open fingers. And also, this technique works better just touching the body gently rather than just off the body.

Practice these pelvic stabilising techniques twice daily if possible or once a day minimum. Do so, last thing at night before retiring. They will also help you sleep. These fluid techniques should only be performed on a sofa or bed or couch, not on the floor.

The energy/fluid drive however, that is, the technique projecting electrical/biological energy can also be performed sitting or standing - you may easily adapt to different bodily positions for this one.

Happily, it is quite possible to practise these STABILIZING techniques by themselves, especially so, if the PELVIC CORRECTION techniques are difficult or impossible to execute. These STABILIZING techniques should balance/correct the pelvis alone - they are powerful, especially if both sides of the pelvis are dealt with as explained.

If you give some thought to it, these Pelvic Correction Techniques may be executed sitting-down. Trying them in this way allows you to do them at work and when travelling.
As long as you can perform the Pelvic Correction Techniques then practice them at least 3 to 4 times a day i.e. throughout the day. These, you may practise on the floor if you wish.

N.B. Book: Craniosacral Therapy by John E. Upledger. V-spread techniques

These Stabilising Techniques are your **'fail-safe' Systems,** especially when you are not sure whether you suffer a 'drop' or a 'twist', and cannot ascertain which dysfunction you have. In other words, exercising one, or both Stabilising Techniques, will re-align your pelvis anyway especially if these techniques are exercised both sides of your body.

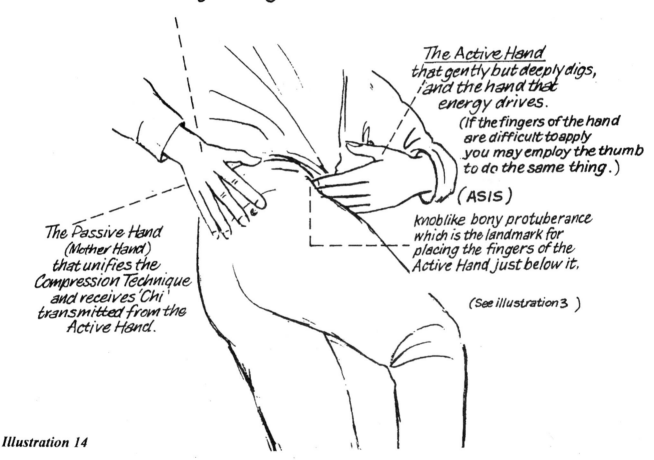

Note: Position this right hand directly over right buttock.

The Active Hand that gently but deeply digs, and the hand that energy drives.
(If the fingers of the hand are difficult to apply you may employ the thumb to do the same thing.)

(ASIS)

knoblike bony protuberance which is the landmark for placing the fingers of the Active Hand just below it.

(See illustration 3)

The Passive Hand (Mother Hand) that unifies the Compression Technique and receives 'Chi' transmitted from the Active Hand.

Illustration 14

Techniques Fluid Compression Drive and Fluid Energy Drive for gaining Pelvic Stability

Illustration 15

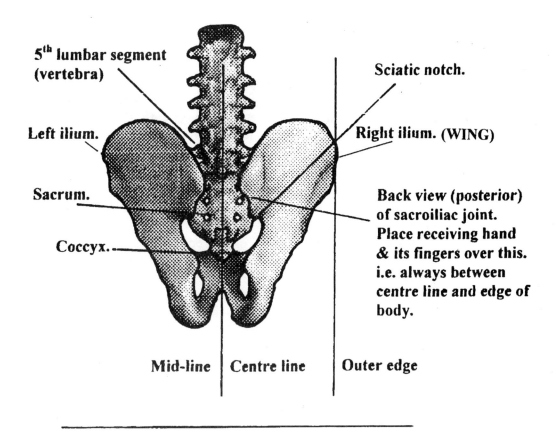

5th lumbar segment (vertebra)

Left ilium.

Sacrum.

Coccyx.

Sciatic notch.

Right ilium. (WING)

Back view (posterior) of sacroiliac joint. Place receiving hand & its fingers over this. i.e. always between centre line and edge of body.

Mid-line | Centre line | Outer edge

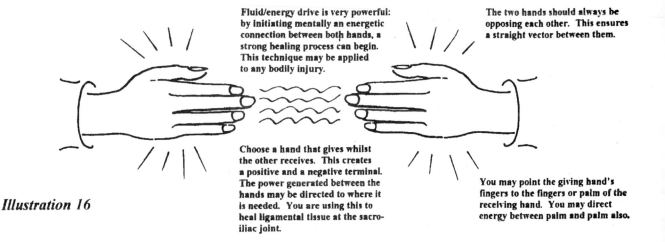

Fluid/energy drive is very powerful: by initiating mentally an energetic connection between both hands, a strong healing process can begin. This technique may be applied to any bodily injury.

The two hands should always be opposing each other. This ensures a straight vector between them.

Choose a hand that gives whilst the other receives. This creates a positive and a negative terminal. The power generated between the hands may be directed to where it is needed. You are using this to heal ligamental tissue at the sacro-iliac joint.

You may point the giving hand's fingers to the fingers or palm of the receiving hand. You may direct energy between palm and palm also.

Illustration 16

TO SUMMARISE THE CONTENTS OF CHAPTER SIX

- Several **Stabilisation Techniques** exist, which may help you to exercise the **Pelvic Correction Techniques** more easily and perhaps these may not be needed as often.
- I recommend the powerful **Fluid Compression Drive.** This technique by itself, not only helps stabilise the pelvis, but also returns the pelvis to its proper balanced state. Even better, the **Thumb Drive Technique.** View Illustration 2, page **7**. This does it both ways as well.
- They may be applied once a day, but twice is even better.
- The Thumb Drive is powerful because you are applying **breath** to stroke/plunge/dig. You may work out any pain, in the location, as indicated.
- The **Fluid/Energy Drive** will be a little difficult for many of you to comprehend, but is powerful.
- It requires the projection of 'chi' or [life/energy].
- It is used in addition with the Fluid Compression Drive technique as indicated, or optionally.
- You have the freedom to choose whichever suits your temperament.
- Both methods should be applied in **Recovery Position**, though this is not essential.

N.B. Book: Craniosacral Therapy by John E. Upledger. V-spread technique

---

THE DREAM

Mind and matter in collusion

Living our dreams in confusion

Acting the dream is but illusion

Time now for the awakened infusion

To bring the dream to its conclusion

C. Kathy Richardson.   January 2001

Chapter Seven

APPLICATION OF ENERGY AS A TOOL FOR HEALING

In addition to the given procedures in the previous chapters, it is recommended, following the execution of all Pelvic Correction work, to rub your lumbar region with the back (dorsal) of your fists, up & down; side-to-side; circularly, and also, percussively.

This will generate kidney and 'Yang Chi' * as well as to bring blood, fluids, and oxygen to that area.   Thus, you are giving yourself a mini-treatment and increasing pelvic stability. See Illustration #17.

- • * 'Chi' (Chinese) or 'Ki' (Japanese) is that interior force we all possess (life/vitality). Some of us can generate more of this 'chi' than others' determined by our inherited physical constitution. It represents the difference between that which is alive and that which is not.

- • Either that mysterious life-force is there in a living thing, or it is not, in which case it is dead, or inanimate.

- • There are differences in the type of 'Chi' that accompanies life, and this helps to engender all the multiplicity of life forms, as well producing varied 'Chi' within a given life form.

- • Generating kidney and 'Yang Chi' [heat] will help the pelvis' stability.

You should be able to enjoy a reduction and possibly an elimination of aches and pains in for instance the back (upper, middle, lower); upper arm; shoulder; neck and knee, providing the pelvis remains aligned. This is because the whole spine is now sitting on an horizontal base (pelvis) rather than an oblique angled one caused by misaligned components belonging to this base. Thus, the whole spine can enjoy absence of strain, erectness and therefore release from any trapped nerves.   Of course, for some of you, the situation may well be more complicated – so many people experience agony when their pelvises are only a tiny bit dislocated; whilst others, who have the same small dislocation, feel hardly a twitch. For most of you though, many benefits will be experienced and enjoyed.

You should also notice more energy and a feeling of well-being. <u>Some minor medical conditions may clear-up:</u> the skeletal frame appreciates being aligned. Since all else within the body is 'slung-on' to this frame, then all else does benefit.

You may rub the lumbar region with the back of your hands made into fists directly on to the bare skin, indeed, I recommend it. The skin will become nice and reddened and loosened, and the whole process could work better.

Illustration 17

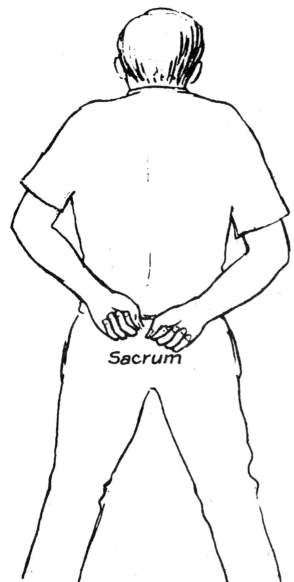

Rub fists up and down
vertically, side to side,
horizontally and
circularly and also
percussively. Hit with
both fists together
as though the fists are
tied to each other
over the central
Sacrum area.

Sacrum

Lumbar-rub Technique

Notes on 'LUMBAR-RUB' TECHNIQUE

- The **Lumbar-Rub Technique** is very valuable, because it indicates to you that you are able, to some extent, to treat yourself therapeutically. Especially so for this, often painful, area of the body.
- You may rub, with the back of your fists, as described on page 38, directly on bare skin, indeed, I recommend it, as this area will become nice and reddened!
- You may use a mixture, of say, 3 essential oils, such as with: Cedarwood, fennel, and ginger, for additional therapeutic purposes. These oils in small quantities dropped into a carrier oil of say, Grapeseed, and dropped-on the back (dorsal) area of your hands, and to be rubbed into your lower lumbar back, as previously described, will nourish the kidneys energetically.
- This kidney association is important as the kidneys energetically rule the bones and joints, among other bodily structures, and it is specific bones and joints that are in question.
- This technique, in addition to receiving particular therapeutic treatments (read page 40), as recommended, and taking-on especial disciplines to improve your general health (read page 41), will give you a sense of achieving your health aims on a number of planes. See pages 42, 43 and 44.

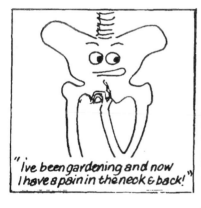

"I've been gardening and now I have a pain in the neck & back!"

Patrick the Pelvis...

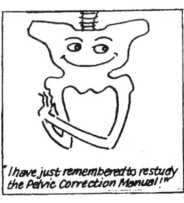

"I have just remembered to restudy the Pelvic Correction Manual!"

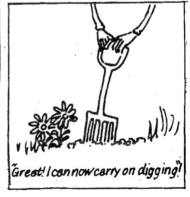

"Great! I can now carry on digging!"

VARIOUS THERAPIES THAT WILL ASSIST PELVIC CORRECTION TECHNIQUES

Now it is the time to consider follow-up treatments that will help further stabilise your pelvis as well as to improve your general health:

Note: Most therapists/doctors will not be familiar with Pelvic Correction. It is therefore personally your responsibility to work with it. These therapists/doctors may assist you however, using their own disciplines and slowly pelvic stability will be gained mostly by default, whatever, you are the one controlling the pelvic alignment.

- Shiatsu
- Acupuncture
- Cranio-sacral therapy
- Osteopathy
- Chiropractic
- Polarity therapy
- Rolfing
- Zero-balancing
- Bowen technique
- Reflexology
- Aromatherapy
- Therapeutic Massage
- And many more types of body therapies - all helpful

Note: You cannot rely on any of these treatments administered and enjoyed, to return the pelvis to its true horizontal position. What is required always, is your direct intervention using the given techniques, and employing optionally, existing osteopaths' and chiropractors' skills. However, any of these therapies will help your body/mind to better health generally.

DISCIPLINES, WHICH WILL IMPROVE HEALTH:

Taking-up seriously, that is, to practise, any of the following disciplines will also help to bring pelvic stability as well as to improve overall health:

- Alexander Technique (no relationship to Alexander Barrie's System)
- Pilates
- Hatha-yoga
- Tai-chi
- Chi-quong
- Other soft or hard-Martial Arts

Important note: *It is more than possible that any of these Systems can move the pelvis 'out of kilter'. Therefore, <u>always end working sessions</u> <u>with the Pelvic Correction Techniques as learned</u>. This also applies to any kind of activity, whether digging in the garden, shifting furniture, running, cycling, pumping iron etc., always finish these activities with your techniques in case your pelvis dislocates when there is exertion/activity.*

In addition and if possible, never stretch that side of the body that suffers a 'drop' to the pelvis. So, if a 'drop' exists on the right side never stretch that side. It is over-stretched anyway. You may stretch the left side of the body, and I recommend it. Stretching the left side of the body in this case may help to correct the right side that suffers a 'drop' to the pelvis. Of course, a left-side 'drop' needs a right-side stretch.

PATIENTS' ATTITUDE MAY INCLUDE:

- Laziness.
- Expect doctor to do all.
- Should be a quick 'fix'.
- The thought of improving health-wise and actually getting well becomes unbearable for some of us. We will not get that sympathy and all else from family, friends, and State!
- Previous drugs and surgical procedures may interfere with progress, and some people will prefer to stay with these anyway.

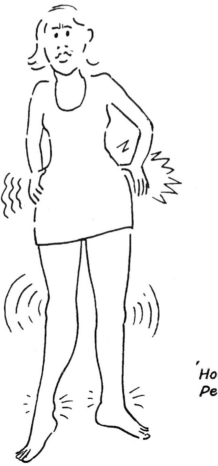

How I felt before Pelvic Correction.

Chapter Eight

POTENTIAL COMPLICATIONS

The following , in a sense, is an additional cogent topic of this manual :

For every 10 people, 5 will suffer a 'twist' or a 'drop', and that is all they will have to contend with, that is, to deal with one or the other dysfunction only.

The other 5 people, which is actually every other person, will diagnose a 'twist' or a 'drop', deal with what they find, say, a 'drop', and a day or two later still be in pain/discomfort. This is because the other lesion the 'twist' now has become prevalent.

The 'twist' lesion is being hidden by the 'drop' lesion, which was first diagnosed. This new lesion is usually on the same side. Occasionally, it is on the opposite side.

It means that the sufferer has now to perform the two techniques, one immediately after the other to obtain pelvic stability.

It is a question of patience, and perspective. If you become pain free, it is well worth the inconvenience of practicing the two techniques one after the other: 'belt and braces'. **Even so, you now have the 'Regulator' to get round this, because this technique should make the Pelvic Correction regardless of the type of lesion involved.**

Bear in mind that you may not have succeeded in performing sufficiently well the technique applied to the result of your first diagnosis, i.e. you may have diagnosed correctly a 'drop' and not applied sufficiently strongly the appropriate technique to neutralize that 'drop'. So, you have to try again more resolutely; and hopefully, you then have only the one technique to perform.

All techniques need to be executed a minimum of 3 times a day at least to obtain the desired results-make them a part of your life, certainly for a year or two or three.

Most people have suffered with back-pain and more for many years, because their pelvis has been 'out of kilter' for many years, so it will take time to reverse this body interior dysfunctional habit.

The truth is that there is no other way - it seems to be a condition of human travail. Even so, persistence, diligence and strength in the execution of these techniques will bring the desired results.

ESSENTIAL GUIDE NOTES:

As you may know, the lower back (lumbar area) may suddenly and unexpectedly give-way causing pain and muscular spasm. Life is disrupted - it happens. Perhaps you the sufferer have moved an object in the wrong way. (Always be square-on to an object when lifting it, see Illustration 18). Perhaps too much is happening in your life right now; whatever, your pelvis has definitely moved 'out of kilter' causing the lumbar problem.

You should rest for a number of days, though even from the beginning, I would advise, that you elect to receive as much back massage as is possible, perhaps from your partner. Any kind of treatment, even in the acute stage will accelerate the healing process.

A given pelvic ilium (wing) may continue to slip over several hours, over several days. Be persistent in your corrective technique work. The output you expect success-wise, depends always on the amount of your input.

Lifting any medium to heavy items __must__ always be performed square-on; otherwise the pelvis may sublux. Never lift an item that is at your side, turn square-on to it, then you can lift it. (View illustration 18)

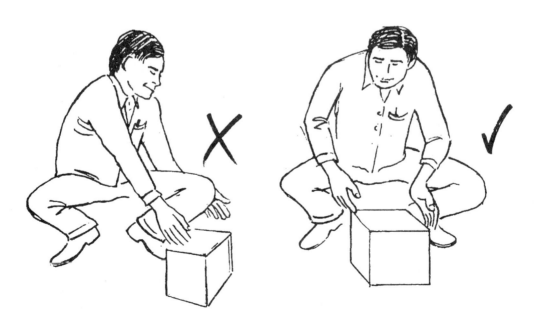

Illustration 18

IMPORTANT ADDITIONAL NOTES:

- You are not really a robotic human. You cannot be perfect and carry out your obligations technique-wise day in day out. When you forget to perform your techniques, the pelvis may slip out-of-kilter, and if it does, it is usually only slight, and you feel this discrepancy, if not in your back then <u>distally in your legs, torso, shoulder, neck or arms.</u> Just return to the techniques in your own time, and pelvic balance will be restored and you will feel better again. You realise you have a great measure of control now.

- It could happen that things are going well for you, and the pelvis is stabilising and then suddenly you are in pain. Your pelvis might now be showing a new problem. Re-diagnose, using the methods previously explained.

- About 1 in 100 people have a true leg length discrepancy even after their pelvises are straightened. These people should have some kind of heel-lift for the shortened leg. If the difference is ¼ inch then the heel lift has to be ¼ inch. It should be transferred from shoe to shoe. The best material for heel-lifts is cork obtained from an osteopathic supplier. See Yellow pages. However, you may improvise with materials, and have heel-lifts for all your shoes for convenience sake. Messrs. Woolworths have rubber heels that can be used satisfactorily.

- A previously fractured leg will usually (but not always) shorten by ¼ inch. Even after pelvic re-alignment, that leg will need a heel lift.

- As already stated after some months of success gaining pelvic stability, unexpectedly for whatever reason the pelvis will move out-of-kilter causing back pain and other problems. These are the times you will put more zeal into your Pelvic Correction Techniques. **However, this action may not work, the pelvis has decided to <u>lock</u> into the wrong position.** This is the time you will require an ABSPC Practitioner or Osteopath or Chiropractor.

- **Sometimes, you may have to perform Pelvic Correction every hour. It happens. For whatever reason, the pelvis just will not stabilise this particular day or this particular week. Eventually it will stabilise, quite often suddenly and unexpectedly, and you may return to normal regular Pelvic Correction times. Hopefully, this sort of anomaly only lasts a few days.**

- Taking the above statement further, if Pelvic Correction is performed immediately following any kind of exertion (sport or work), back disorders may be avoided.

- You cannot really do harm with the techniques in this manual, they go with the flow and not against it. Even when the pelvis is already aligned, the techniques can still be performed. Some patients may panic, after practicing certain procedures things seem to go terribly wrong. You need to be re-assured that these techniques just need more time and more zeal with their practice.

- Generally speaking, you should aim to straighten the whole spine after Pelvic Correction. If not, then <u>rotated segments (distorted vertebrae)</u> can work downwards to undo the pelvis' stability, though not always: it is possible for the spine to straighten itself, but seeking help for this is recommended.

- Any kind of exercise regimen is beneficial provided the techniques for Pelvic Correction are added on at the end of an exercise session <u>immediately.</u> It will take 6 months to a year or two to settle the pelvis. Some people do well straight away; others take much, much longer time for this.

- You should visit an Osteopath, Chiropractor or an ABSPC Practitioner to help make more concrete your progress in Pelvic Correction. **You yourself can look after your pelvis.** The professionals can do the other bits. The 'mental thing' may be crucial here. Do you have an **attitude** problem? Do you lack self-esteem? All this may be relevant to Pelvic Correction. Psychotherapy is then recommended or even better: read Brandon Bays 'The Journey' and 'Conversations With God' by Neale Donald Walsch.

- It is important to get-up off the couch, bed or floor following Pelvic Correction. Walk up and down the room to enable blood, fluids, oxygen, Chi and any other entity yet to be discovered, to flow through the body and especially so, within the pelvic area. After a minute or two, you should walk as a true homo-sapiens and not as Neanderthal man.

- Your original discomfort in the lower back does not always cease immediately, that may take another 36 hours to happen. However, you are empowered, and will not feel that hopelessness that you felt before you came to this. So too other aches and pains may not cease immediately.

- Never put a wallet or any other item of thickness into your back trouser pocket. As you sit on it, it will distort the pelvis. Men-folk are guilty of this especially when in motorcars. So the more money you put into your wallet the more back-pain!!!

- **It is not possible to suffer a 'drop' or a 'twist' at the same moment in time – it is either one or the other at a given moment.**

The pelvis is the **FOUNDATION OF THE SKELETAL FRAME** and when it moves out-of-kilter, the segments of the whole spine can be affected badly. Re-aligning the whole spine, if necessary, better ensures that the pelvis stabilises*. Being the foundation of the skeletal frame makes it also the FOUNDATION FOR THE ABDOMINAL CONTENTS: *'HARA' (Hara: see next page).*

* To be treated by an Osteopath, Chiropractor or ABSPC Practitioner.

A healthy 'Hara' will assist your strength, endurance, and stability on many levels, including potential spiritual grace. Better health can also be enjoyed when your 'centre of gravity area – <u>Hara' is truly centred helped by sitting on a firm and aligned base (the pelvis).</u>

At best, you can act and think from this place (Hara) of 'being' as its energy and power radiate outwards and permeate all cellular and molecular structures. The illusion of separateness from all and everything can to a large extent be lessened when you are centred here, because this inner-self perceives the connectivity of everything.

POLITICAL CANDIDNESS:

Finally, I would advise you choose to recondition yourself to think in terms of **self-help**, if you have not already. By taking responsibility for your body now, it [the body] will serve you well to enable you to discover in this life *your true self.* The awareness you will gain from practising this System will be for many of you the beginning of health/spiritual quest; even an epiphany.

Individuals, who say they cannot find time to execute the recommended techniques, could be harming themselves. Less time in the local Public House, and less time looking at television will supply the minutes required.

Even so, it is easily possible to practise all techniques while actually watching T.V. and even in the Public House, at the workplace also. Most techniques given may be applied sitting down. They only have to be adapted, and they will work 90% of the time when carried-out diligently.

By all means, visit an Osteopath, or Chiropractor or both, but also an ABSPC Practitioner if possible for further treatment. However, <u>your job</u> is to look after your pelvis, and you will then observe and experience that osteopathic/chiropractic treatment will work superbly.

Chapter Nine

SCIATICA:

Sciatica seems to have acquired mystical status as to its manifestation. The problem is a simple one. Once the pelvis is stabilised, sciatic pain at side or back of thigh begins to disappear in most cases. This includes any pain/discomfort at the pubic bone and/or groin area and lower back, though, a great deal of local bodywork at the groin area may be needed initially. Speaking of which, please bear in mind that although the **origin** of most musculo-skeletal aches and pains are from a dysfunctional pelvis, **you should still employ some sort of bodywork on the local painful areas: shoulder for example; and the spine itself, ideally, should be re-aligned osteopathically.** (Read Spine Versus Pelvis page 14)

However, it is not erroneous to think that all the various medical conditions mentioned above, are actually symptoms of one problem only, namely: a dysfunctional pelvis.

On the great sciatic nerve, a word further:

When an ilium (wing of pelvis) has 'dropped' or 'twisted', as driven by some of the dysfunctional components of the pelvis, it will often have a direct ill-affect on the sciatic *rami* (original branches which go to form the great sciatic nerve), especially because, these branches pass through the **Great Sciatic Notch.** See illustration 5a. & 6.

This **sciatic notch**, which is a component of the posterior (back) of the *ilium,* moves out of its normal position and thus leans and impinges into these *rami.* Hence, pain ensues, often along the length of the sciatic nerve itself.

In addition, these sciatic nerves are pulled and stretched in this area, and may give rise also to sciatic pain. It is true that, following a prolapsed, or worse, an herniated disc (slipped disc) at say between L3 and L4 (View Illustration 7), the soft contents of the cartilaginous disc having ruptured and spilled-out, that this may also impinge on the nerve-fibres that make an exit/entry at between L3 and L4, and thus have a direct malefic affect on these sciatic nerve fibres.

Though sciatica may be lessened as the pelvis is corrected and **lumbar segments re-aligned,** there may be discomfort still; and until some other form of healing takes-place, such as with rest taken by the sufferer, and gentle back massage/healing, or at worst corrective surgery, will the sciatic pain disappear. View Illustrations 6. & 7.

This manual is not intended to usurp or replace the skills implemented by Osteopaths and Chiropractors. It merely gives you 'rule of thumb' techniques that work 95% of the time.

PELVIC CORRECTION IN RELATION TO PREGNANCY

In the round, correcting the pelvis during pregnancy is favourable. The safest time of all administering the relevant techniques is during the second trimester. Other safe times, only slightly less so, are during the first and the third trimester. The importance here is to apply common sense and gentleness when executing the technique or techniques.

Your baby [foetus] will enjoy its own development inside a womb that is upright and level (vertical and horizontal): only possible with an aligned pelvis.

A pelvis which is in-kilter, allows better fluid and blood and 'chi' movement for the whole abdominal cavity and its visceral components, rendering not only proper growth for the foetus, but better health for the bearer (mother).

It is, unfortunately, not as yet recognised sufficiently that a dysfunctional pelvis, so commonplace, contributes to the multiplicity of pathological problems, physical and psychological, a woman may experience before, during, and after pregnancy, because this state of things engenders difficulties such as with potential: organ prolapse, hernias, deficient blood/oxygen supply, deficient absorption of nutrients via intestines, and many more disorders also involving bladder and bowel control. These of course adversely affect mother and child.

Hopefully, in time, it will be a matter of routine to re-align, and to stabilise pelvises of pregnant mothers.

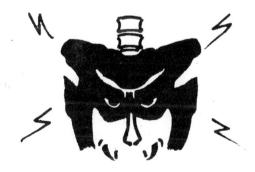

Helvis the Pelvis

It is worthy of some research, but on observation, I have noticed that Inguinal Hernia in men, and Femoral Hernia in women, almost without exception, manifest on the same body side as that of an osseous prolapse [*drop*] of the pelvis. That is, a downward inferior-tilt, side to side. Usually, right-side downwards (inferior), but not always.

Naturally, with a pelvis out-of-kilter, in this case, an actual '*drop*' on the right side, and making the leg on that side *apparently* longer than its partner leg. Existing over a period of time, there would be a continuous stretching of fascia at the right groin area.

Since we are writing about the chronic dislocation of the pelvis, which has been thus over a substantial number of years, and because the pelvis has not been re-aligned, various layers of **fascial** tissue will have a tendency to tear, engendering **hernial** proclivities.

Pelvic dislocation, so commonplace, is responsible for a number of visceral prolapsus. A common side-to-side tilt of the pelvis, will definitely push the abdominal contents to one side, perhaps only fractionally, but still be an irritant to the fascia, and especially to the visceral [organ] contents below the umbilicus as well as above the umbilicus.

If there is a right side '*drop*' to the pelvis, the right kidney will be forced downwards (inferiorly), if only by a few millimetres. This downward tendency of the right kidney will have an adverse affect on the liver structurally, which in turn, will have a downward pull on the diaphragm on that side, and so it goes on through the right lung and to the shoulder (clavicle). This shoulder then develops a different height to its partner shoulder (clavicle).

I have noticed common conditions such as with indigestion ceasing to be, when the skeletal frame has been re-aligned, with emphasis on correction of pelvic subluxation.

Of course, if there is a left-side '*drop*', all the anomalies above will be engendered on the opposite side of the body, and that would include spleen and stomach organs.

All visceral organs have their own intelligence. If they are forced to move, if only fractionally from their normal placings, they become increasingly sensitive, but pathologically so.

If a given organ is already operating deficiently or be deranged in any way, it will be aggravated, and its ill-effects on the bodily system experienced more keenly!

RESTLESS/IRRITABLE LEG SYNDROME

This curious condition is uncommon, but is felt nevertheless by the sufferer as somewhat pestilential.

The legs seem to have a life of their own, especially when the owner of these legs is incumbent. What develops are sensations of tickling, burning, prickling and aching and a strong desire to get-up and move around, which is perhaps for many the only way of dealing with this peculiar compulsion.

Most often there is writhing, straining, and moving of the lower limbs and especially the calves, ankles and feet, from which these queer compulsions arise.

Some people benefit from cooling their legs, others from warming them. Even so, we know that a reduction of caffeine, alcohol, and, abstinence from smoking will reduce this irritation.

The condition also engenders restless sleep, as the lower legs want to move incessantly. Of course this will be tiresome for the sleeping partner, assuming one is there!

The intensity of the problem varies from person to person, and the more restless/intense that problem is, may well affect the mental state of the sufferer, manifesting in a particular form of depression.

There are several common threads with those who suffer this syndrome.

1. Invariably their pelvises are subluxed/dislocated. This naturally leads to poor circulation of blood and fluids into the legs, including the retardation of certain neural pathways in that vicinity. From the oriental point of view 'chi' is partially prevented in travelling through its normal channels.

   STABILISE THE PELVIS BY RE-ALIGNMENT, AND A REDUCTION OF THE INTENSITY OF RESTLESS LEG SYNDROME WILL BE ENJOYED. IN ADDITION, WITH AN INCREASED FLOW OF THOSE PRODUCTS INTO THE LEGS, AS MENTIONED ABOVE, THE LEG STRUCTURES WILL BE NOURISHED, AS SKELETAL ALIGNMENT IS MAINTAINED.

2. Look to the **liver** and the **gall bladder**. These organs, and in particular their energetic aspects, rule the sinews (ligaments and tendons) from the oriental medicine point of view. It is probable that the tendons are not sufficiently supplied with liver blood. This may cause contractions, affecting muscle and sinew.

   As liver **'chi'** is deficient, the **smooth actions** of various organic structures and especially those in the lower limbs, in this instance, are adversely affected, and thus irritation follows in that area.

51

3. It has been known for years now that in The Western-world, certainly, the soils are almost depleted of many essential minerals. Minerals, which are necessary for we humans to exist in life in a healthy way. An absence of particular minerals in our diet usually leads to a number of deficiencies affecting our physiology, especially in the form of **tics** of one sort or another.

I HAVE OBSERVED THAT WITH THE USE OF <u>COLOIDAL MINERALS</u>, MINERALS THAT CAN BE ABSORBED PROPERLY BY THE BODY, THERE MAY BE A SUBSTANTIAL REDUCTION IN THE IRRITABLE LEG PROBLEM. I WOULD RECOMMEND THE CONSUMPTION OF THIS TYPE OF PRODUCT, RATHER THAN IN ANY OTHER FORM.

From the point of view of Astrological Medicine the most common Zodiacal Signs involved in this syndrome are **Sagittarius** and **Aquarius,** and to some extent **Pisces.** This does not mean to say that people have to own these heavenly archetypes by **Sun Sign.** What matters, is if there is some emphasis within one or all of these signs, because these signs are occupied by two or more planets, as indicated in an individual natal chart.

The signs: **Sagittarius** and **Pisces** are, by tradition ruled by the great planet **Jupiter.** Symbolically, Sagittarius being its residence during the day whilst [he] occupies his nights in the Pisces Mansion. (This interpretation is symbolical).

Jupiter rules, amongst other things, the **liver** and the **gall bladder** from the Chinese Astrology point of view in that both are given to the **'Wood'** element. The meaning of **'wood'** in relation to human life means: just as a tree in its magnificence thrusts upwards and outwards, so does **'wood'** within us, compelling us in varying degrees to venture forth with energy and enterprise, enthusiasm and curiosity. The thirst for knowledge through exploration is often overwhelming, engendering the need to keep our body/mind/spirit open, inquisitive, and moving. Especially so, if in your natal chart there is an emphasis with the three signs mentioned above.

These are Jovian principles acting interiorly within humanity, whether it [humanity] likes it or not; and especially so, again, if the three signs mentioned above are prevalent. The power of the 'wood'; element is present in all of us anyway. The more a human recognises this gift within him/her the freer he/she is and the more successful mundanely and hopefully, in time, spiritually. It is this energy compulsion that may go awry physiologically, and help to bring-on the restless leg problem. This is because of a potential innate uncontrollable desire to go walking/exploring without due purpose.

The **Aquarian Sign** in other traditions is ruled by Chronos, the great planet **Saturn.** However, there are mixed connections to this restless leg syndrome with this planet, and nothing certain.   With the god Zeus (Jupiter) however, there is certainty, as outlined above. A correspondence may be made though, through the ruling of **the Aquarian Sign** to the **gall bladder** (see above), as indicated in Chinese Medicine/Astrology.

The sign **Aquarius** in other traditions is also given to the **Air Element.** This will link it definitely to **Vata Dosha*** as in **Ayurvedic Medicine** theory and practice. **Vata** rules energetically all of the body **from below the umbilicus.** And we know that excess **Vata** will produce abnormal movements. Excess movements will, in this case, manifest in an almost impossible capacity to remain still legwise.

WHEN BEING TREATED BY AN AYURVEDIC PHYSICIAN. HE/SHE WILL RECOMMEND AN ADJUSTMENT TO THE DIET, ADVISING WHICH FOODS TO AVOID AND ESPECIALLY THOSE FOODS TO SIDESTEP, WHICH EXCITE 'VATA DOSHA', BECAUSE MANY TYPES OF FOOD INCREASE THE 'VATA DOSHA' AFFECT, MAKING IT EVEN MORE UNSTABLE IN ACTION. OTHER DEVICES WILL BE RECOMMENDED TO REDUCE THE 'VATA' AFFECT. IT WILL ALSO BE RECOMMENDED TO EAT THOSE FOODS THAT HELP TO INCREASE THE POWER OF THE REMAINING TWO DOSHAS, THEREBY CREATING A GREATER BALANCE IN THE INDIVIDUAL ON ALL LEVELS. THIS SHOULD MEAN ALSO A REDUCTION IN THE RESTLESS LEG PROBLEM.

What is written above should help the reader to see the wider view of this particular condition.

* For understanding Vata Dosha principles, any book on Ayurvedic Medicine will convey the various meanings. Also, see author's note on Ayurvedic Doshas In Relation To The Pelvis next.

THE INDIAN AYURVEDIC DOSHAS IN RELATION TO THE PELVIS:

Ref: *dosha* (singular) is the Sanskrit name given to any one of the three main human types, with specific propensities: ***kapha; pitta; and vata.*** (***doshas.*** plural)

<u>Briefly</u>, *kapha* types: **are well-built large frame, strong, unhurried and graceful, reliable, consistant, stable. Endomorph. Practical in thought and action. Cautious.** *Kapha* **originates from the lower abdomen, pelvic contents, and legs. However, the body parts: stomach organ; lung; chest; neck and head, basically means that** *kapha* **is** <u>resident</u> **energetically in the upper body parts. (See next page).**

Pitta **types: are medium build. Mesomorph. Good shape, enterprising, run-the-show, driven, sharp, hot, clever. Have a vision. Body parts: small intestine; liver; gall bladder and spleen. Centred in middle part of body: epigastric region.**

Vata **types: are usually thin or wiry, short or very tall. Ectomorph. Mutable, excitable, many interests, creative, vague, academic and not always practical, centred somewhat in the head. Always on the move: restless.** *Vata* **originates from the chest, neck and head. However, body parts: colon; bladder; pelvis; genitalia and legs, basically means that** *vata* **is** <u>resident</u> **energetically in the lower body parts. (See next page)**

*This division of three, actually, may be seen in all aspects of creation. For anything in life to exist, whether animal, vegetable or mineral in origin, must be subject to **The Law of Three**: Active (pitta) **Passive** (kapha) and **Neutral** (vata). It is applied also to the three divisions of the body. And those are: upper, middle, and lower. This supplies us with a wider understanding of the underlying meaning of the Triple Heater or Triple Burner as taught in Traditional Chinese Medicine; in that, the Triple Heater relates amongst other things to the balance or imbalance of the three doshas to one another and their relational effects, in the human body. Most of us have an emphasis in our natures in any one or two of the doshas.*

The pelvis is considered as belonging to ***vata dosha*** - as one of its components.

This implies that ***vata***, resident in the lower body including legs, **energetically** influences the health of the structures of the lower body, from the umbilicus downwards, and in particular the **pelvis.**

We would not be wrong in concluding therefore that **pelvic instability, which is mostly at the root of back-pain**, is engendered by a ***vata-dosha*** problem/imbalance. And this is true.

However, in my experience with Pelvic Correction over the years, all *doshic* types suffer equally with pelvic instability/dislocation. That is, both *pitta* and *kapha* types are equally not immune to pelvic subluxation.

In one respect this agrees with Ayurvedic pathology in, that it is stated: "that a prolonged imbalance in any one *dosha* will definitely adversely affect the remaining two doshas in due course". That is, there is a morbid migration of material, and imbalance from one body site onto/into another body site at a progressive stage in a given pathology. Of course, and in addition, a given *dosha* may be constitutionally deficient or overly dominant, and this situation will produce the same adverse effect as stated above.

I wish to proffer an important factor in Ayurveda — seemingly, not put into the texts of books on Ayurvedic medicine, as follows:

To understand the following, it is necessary to have a basic comprehension of *yin/yang*, as expounded in oriental literature/medicine. **The basic law of life is that:**

<u>Yin</u> attracts <u>Yang</u> and visa versa.

<u>Yang</u> is: heat, light, heaven, space. <u>Yin</u> is: cool, dark, earth, boundaries.

<u>Yang</u>, is consonant with the <u>air</u> and <u>ether</u> elements as well as the upper and middle body *Chakras*. All from heaven and *Yang*, and may be associated therefore with the *Vata dosha* which is rooted in the upper body.

<u>Yin</u>, is consonant with the earth and water elements as well as the lower body *Chakras*. All from earth and *Yin*, and may be associated therefore with the *Kapha dosha* which is rooted in the lower body.

<u>Then why are the upper parts of the body given to *Kapha* and the lower parts of the body given to *Vata*, as taught by the ancient *Rishis*?</u>

Because, as a magnet orientates to magnetic north with its south pole only [the magnet itself], you have: yin and yang attract and heaven and earth attract and positive and negative attract, then the lower body which is basically represented by earth and water elements and associated with earth, will attract heaven, bringing it downwards, or *Vata energetically to dwell in the lower body.*

And, the upper body, which is basically represented by air and ether and associated with heaven and light, will attract earth bringing it upwards, or *Kapha energetically to dwell in the upper body.*

Indeed, *Yang/Vata* must have a downward movement and *Yin/Kapha* must have an upward movement. Each to attract the other. *Pitta (fire)* is in the middle stabilising/regulating the other two.

<u>The statements above may help to explain this Ayurvedic paradox to an extent.</u>

SUPPLEMENTARY SECTION ON 'MUSCLE ENERGY TECHNIQUES'
(These MET's have a Japanese *Sotai** bent, and therefore they are not strictly MET's)

These additional procedures are based on the common occurrence of the shortening/spasm of two separate muscles namely: Psoas and Piriformis. Both are paired in that there are two Psoas and two Piriformis muscles. A good anatomical atlas will place the Psoas as being deep inside the rear aspect of the abdomen, and the piriformis as deep within the buttock behind the Gluteus Maximus.

It appears that these two muscles, more than other muscles, are especially affected adversely by all of human travail, including life stress and negative emotion. These happenings, on the mundane plane, bedevil our lives interiorly and therefore exteriorly, and tend to have an affect via the 'spleen' on these particular muscles whose manifestation thus, is usually a self shortening, self tightening or a self weakening.

When the left-side psoas shortens, it may lead to a 'drop' right side, and vice versa.
When the left-side piriformis shortens, it may lead to a 'twist' right side, and vice versa

The point of this argument is to indicate that in addition to previous explanations in this manual as to why our pelvises dislocate, these muscles are often culpable and therefore involved.

It is recommended therefore to practice, say once a day, one of the following techniques according to whether you suffer a 'twist' or a 'drop' lesion.

FOR THE 'DROP':

1. If you have a right-side 'drop', <u>push left flexed leg</u> (bent at knee) away from you but do not allow it to move away from you by clasping with your hands the underside of the thigh. (If with a left 'drop' push right flexed leg)
2. Hold in this way for a count of 12 (2 counts a second) with the in-breath held as well.
3. Repeat 4 more times.
4. This will help to tone-up and to correct the left Psoas muscle and therefore it will assist to stabilise the pelvis.

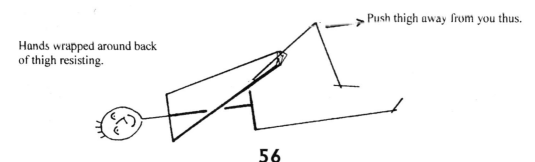

Push thigh away from you thus.

Hands wrapped around back of thigh resisting.

FOR THE 'TWIST':

1. If you have a right-side 'twist', then push the flexed left leg (bent/flexed at the knee) sideways against an object, like the wall. Keep yourself steady and stable on the floor. (If a left 'twist' push flexed right leg)
2. Hold in this way for a count of 12 (2 counts a second) with the in-breath held as well.
3. Repeat 4 more times.
4. This will help to tone-up and correct the left Piriformis muscle and therefore it will assist to stabilise the pelvis.

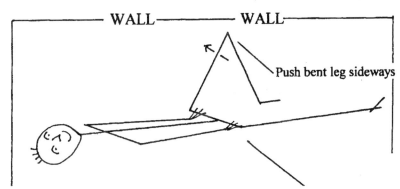

WALL————— WALL

Push bent leg sideways

Hold pelvis steady with both hands thus

* SOTAI (Natural Exercises) by Keizo Hashimoto. ISBN 0-918860-36-9

Appendices:

ESSENTIAL GUIDE NOTES TO HELP MAINTAIN PELVIS AND SPINE:

ACID/ALKALINE BALANCE IN THE BODY

Most of us eat more acid producing foods than alkaline producing foods, such as to create excess acid in the body fluids as a result. This is potentially dangerous because it means that acid build-up enters the joints, bones, ligaments, tendons and muscles. The body cannot eliminate the excess onslaught of acid residues fast enough and therefore pushes this acid excess to where it does least damage and so it sends it to the structures (indicated above) that begin to deteriorate over time. This malefic affect manifests mainly in the:

- **Mesentery** – so the abdomen begins to sag and protrude, and this pulls inwards, anteriorly, the lumbar segments of the spine helping to cause the common lordosis; this lordosis will have a detrimental affect on the remaining spinal segments weakening the skeletal frame. Prolapsed organs are also an important feature to consider with the weakening of the abdominal cavity.
- **The bony spinal segments** - will contract such as to lessen in size their small openings (foramen) at the root of their spinal processes, having a gripping affect on the nerve fibres exiting from these root openings of the spinal processes, and this will cause local pain as well as sciatic problems further along the system.
- **Intervertebral discs** - will contract and harden lessening mobility of spine contributing to stiffness as well as engendering the probability of the rupturing a given disc (slipped-disc).
- **Muscles** – some muscles will become too flaccid engendering hyper-mobility of joints, whilst others will become too tight and stiffened, placing extra strain on joints, enough in fact to dislocate them – especially weight-bearing joints as at the sacro-iliac of the pelvis.
- **Ligaments** – When the body sends excess acid to these, they become dangerously weak and brittle and thus distortion of joints is inevitable, including all vertebral joints of the spine.
- **Osteoporosis** – Acid will leach out of the body mineral calcium, and with the bones especially – this element is an essential ingredient in bone construction.

To avoid these potential problems as much as is possible, it is recommended you lessen the intake of **sweet,** (biscuits, cake, ice-cream sweets etc.,) and **sour** foods, but especially sweet foods, and increase the **consumption of vegetables especially root vegetables and grains.** Lessen the intake of yogurts and fruits as well as meat, fish and fowl. The vegetables should be **organic,** as vegetables from other sources will produce excess acid in your body – as these are contaminated with various toxic chemicals; which is the way virtually all food is cultivated nowadays. Salad items may be acid producing! Drinking mineral water helps to dilute the acid, but no more than 2 litres a day should be consumed as there will be too much strain on the kidney function, and, water puts-out fire – the interior fire of life!

Picture the spine as a spring that can be bent in all directions on all sides and capable of expansion and contraction both ends. This is your spine; the intervertebral discs are the springs, held in tension by specialised ligaments holding the bony segments together with these spring discs in between them.

It is this picture and the actuality that allows the professionals to make safe adjustments to this 'spring'.

By choosing a form of exercise, preferably: 'Yoga' or 'Tai Chi' or 'Chi Kung' or Alexander Technique or 'Pilates', which, within reason, bends and contorts this 'spring', you are loosening any acid residues and certain types of sediment trapped within these structures of the spine (spring). You are also assisting the body's capacity to eliminate these residues helping to maintain a healthy spine.

In addition to 'workouts', it will be understood now why any kind of massage on the spine is beneficial, the most powerful therapy probably: Shiatsu, will definitely 'do the business' though it is not surprising that the recipient of this mode of healing might suffer a re-action the following day. Toxic residues coming away, so to speak, have to do so via the liver and small intestine, and therefore, in this way of exiting, headaches and other forms of discomfort may manifest, but only for a few hours at worst.

SMOKING

It has been proven scientifically that smoking, and this has to include 'pot', causes the fine network of blood vessels in the vertebral segments to contract. This is unfortunate, as the way to keep the intervertebral discs healthy and springy is by their reception of nourishment from those adjacent vertebral segments. The narrowing of these blood vessels disables this process of nourishing, and so the intervertebral disc suffers and the spine deteriorates.

When a person stands-up, a natural compression of the intervertebral discs takes place, and when a person lies-down, these discs swell to receive there necessary nourishment of various fluids directly from the adjacent spinal segments. Therefore, in addition to your regular night's sleep, it is recommended you try to find a time and place during the day to 'siesta' or just to lie-down. The health of the spine will improve as well as the other benefits you will enjoy from a short or long rest during the day.

Hanging upside-down will now be seen as greatly beneficial, so too, allowing the body to dangle when suspended from the hands gripping some means of fixed support well off the ground.

Most of us suffer with Candida Fungus either more, or less. The body's immune system cannot always keep this parasitic entity under control, let alone kill it. This interior pestilence accounts for so much of our mental, emotional and physical health that it may be considered a form of plague.

It is responsible for many of our food allergies, including abnormal re-actions to those entities such as with pollen.

Its greatest concentration of destruction seems to be within the colon, there are other bodily hideouts, but the colon is the main place of residence for this ogre.

If we eat more sweet stuffs than the body can metabolise, we are definitely feeding this 'curse'. This is unfortunate for us, because **the health of the intestine determines, to a large extent, the health of the pelvis,** and **a pelvis that is continually <u>unstable</u>** may well point to a weak intestine.

Probably the most natural form of control for Candida is the consumption of garlic. However, it is probably unwise to eat garlic in its natural state, and in great quantities unless cooked, as it will produce flatulence and diarrhoea, even if not eaten in excess - not to mention the production of excessive heat giving rise skin rashes and much discomfort for some people.

The best way to consume garlic is by taking good quality garlic pills whose content will definitely find its way to the large bowel, killing the Candida in its wake.

WALLET SCIATICA & CHILLY WEATHER

As I have stated in my manual: putting a wallet into your back pocket should be avoided, because as you sit, the horizontality of the pelvis is seriously compromised – there is abnormal pressure against the piriformis muscle also, and all of this has to contribute to pelvic misalignment.

Keep the belly and the lumbar region of the back covered at all times as well as to keep them **warm.** The kidneys **loathe** coldness, and their efficient functioning is vital for healthy bones. Avoid getting them chilled [kidneys], especially with the seasonal changes.

Lifting any weighty object must be performed without a twisting motion - always be square-on to the object you lift, and you will avoid your back giving-way.

ACID – ALKALINE PRODUCING FOODS

Science has divided foods, just as with chemicals, into two value classes:

- Alkaline forming foods   (These are considered safe for consumption)
- Acid forming foods   (These are considered unsafe for consumption if in excess)

If you eat more than 80% alkaline produce, you preserve the normal alkalinity of body fluids that is favourable to health. If you eat more than 20% acid producing foods, your body fluids may become out-of–balance engendering health dangers, both physical and psychological.

ALKALINE (Ideally up to 80% consumption):

Fruits: Apples; Apricots; Avocados; Ripe Bananas; All Berries; Carob Pod; Cherries; Currents; Dates; Figs; Grapes; Mangoes; All Melons; Fresh Olives; Papayas; Peaches; Pears; Raisins; Lemons & Limes.

Vegetables: Ripe Asparagus; Green Beans; Lima Beans; Sprouts; Beets & Tops; Broccoli; Red & White Cabbage; Carrots; Celery; Cauliflower; Chard; Chicory; Chives; Cucumber; Dandelion Greens; Dill; Dock; Dulse; Seaweeds; Endive; Garlic; Kale; Lettuces; Most Mushrooms; Parsnips; Green & Red Peppers; All Potatoes; Pumpkin; Radish; Swede; Sorrel; Soybean; Spinach; Spring Greens; Squash; Turnip & Tops; Watercress.

Dairy Products: Acidophilus; Buttermilk; Raw Milk; Goats Milk; Goats Yogurt.

Flesh Foods: None.

Cereals: Millet; Green Corn (only first 24 hours).

Nuts: Almonds; Roasted Chestnuts; Fresh Coconut.

Miscellaneous: Agar-agar; Alfalfa Products; Coffee Substitutes; Dried Ginger; Honey; Kelp; Tisanes; Mint; Clover; Alfalfa; Sage; Apple Cider Vinegar.

Fresh air, exercise, rest & sleep have an alkalizing affect on the fluids of the body. So too: pleasure, laughter, good conversation, enjoyment and 'love'.

ACID (Ideally no more than 20% consumption):

Fruits: Citrus Fruits; All Preserves; Jellies; Canned, Sugared & Glazed Fruits; Green Bananas; Cranberries; Plums; Prunes and Prune Juice; Non Fresh Olives, Pickles.

Vegetables: Asparagus Tips; All Dried Beans; Brussel Sprouts; Chickpeas; Lentils; Onions; Peanuts; Rhubarb; Tomatoes.

Dairy Products: Butter; All Cheeses; Cottage & Cream Cheese; Ice Cream; Custards; Ices; Milk Boiled, cooked, dried, pasteurized and canned; Eggs.

Flesh Foods: All Meat; Fowl; All Fish; Beef Tea; Shellfish; Gelatine; Gravies.

Cereals: All Flour Products; Buckwheat; Barley; All kinds of Breads; Cakes; Corn; Cornmeal; Flakes; Crackers; All Biscuits; Doughnuts, Dumplings; Macaroni; Spaghetti; Noodles; Oatmeal; Pies & Pastry; Rice; Rye Crisp.

Nuts: All Nuts, and more acidic if Roasted; Dried Coconut; Peanuts.

Miscellaneous: All Alcohol; Cocoa; Chocolate; Flavourings; Marmalades; Preservatives; Tobacco; Condiments; Vinegar; Dressings; Sauces; and drugs; Coffee; Coca Cola.

Acidifiers change the mood for the worst and therefore encourage: worry, fear, anger, hatred, envy, selfishness, greed, and gossip. (The Seven Deadly Sins!). In addition, a more acid body interior is engendered by lack of sleep, overwork, tension, jealousy and resentment.

Actually, there is no food substance that has an absolute value. The foods mentioned above are only for guidance, and anyway, some people need more acid producing foods according to their 'type'. For those who wish to take these lists further, log-on to: www.betterbones.com/alkaline/articles/chart%20p12.pdf

UNDERSTANDING THE EFFECTS OF RECEIVING ALTERNATIVE MEDICAL TREATMENTS – PARTICULARLY THEIR AFTERMATH

- There is no quick-fix, so to speak, to health recovery; even though we have been conditioned in modern times by the orthodox medical profession, that says, following surgery or absorbing a particular allopathic pill: all will be well!

- Re-actions to bodywork will be experienced, particularly following the first and second treatments. There takes place a form of detoxification in the body and mind, and this is an uncomfortable process, but a necessary one.

- Alternative medical effects may be profound and produce unwanted emotions long suppressed. These may always be discussed with the Therapist concerned.

- Importantly, it is to be understood that perhaps as many as six treatments may be needed to turn the first corner as regards progress in health increase, especially so, when in the past, both recent and historical, many prescribed allopathic medicines have been imbibed for specific maladies, and as a consequence have driven the malady deeper into the body – this is common!

- Kindly remember, the allopathic drug course you have taken has dealt with the symptom and not the cause.

It is without doubt that when we suffer any form of illness, condition, or even being 'out of sorts', that our energetic/life-force level is at a low-ebb. This life-force deficiency is probably the first manifestation of an illness, an illness yet to come into being!

In truth, a balanced life full of wholesome habits, uncontaminated thinking and feeling, harmonious surroundings, maintains and indeed increases health. So difficult to acquire, yet we know intuitively what to do, and what to take, to attain, what some would call our natural inheritance.

We have to rid ourselves, mainly of stupidity to enjoy even a modicum of those items mentioned above, but we have to start from somewhere.

Life described in modern times as just a group of chemicals is perhaps the most appalling and damaging mistake of thinking of the present day. The sacredness and the mystery of life have been squeezed into oblivion, causing confusion in all departments of existence and interestingly dismantling: commonsense. This attitude is especially so, in the Western World – is it any wonder why there exists here so much neurosis and consequent psychosis

POST TREATMENT RE-ACTION FOLLOWING THE APPLICATION OF ALTERNATIVE MEDICINE

Curiously, not much is written about post-treatment re-actions patients may suffer. Perhaps it is because we practitioners do not readily acknowledge after treatment discomfort and unease - it might reflect a treatment we administered as incompetent.

We should be guardedly delighted when a patient suffers a re-action, because in most cases it means that we have mobilized those interior body elements that will contribute to a favourable physiological change: rehabilitation may now be possible.

Many 'alternative' therapies engender a re-action as a result of administering their remedies first time round for a given ailment. These re-actions usually do not exceed beyond the first three treatments. A process of detoxification is always in progress within these first healing protocols.

Dividends in the form of physiological progress should follow as the treatments help to push and pull the body systems back into balance - balance being the operative word.

Homeopathic post re-actions are expected, and happen normally within 24 hours. Herbal administrations re-act over several days, as do the more energetic type therapies such as with Acupuncture. Japanese Shiatsu may have a 7day cycle for its action to be complete.

Altogether, the excitation of the body's physiological system, the visceral functions, muscles, sinews, fascia, nerves, fluids and other structures, is favourable, to engender a necessary change not only for the physical body but also for the 'etheric' body, so called.

Toxic body sediment dislodged by treatment will make an exit, amongst other organs, via the Liver and Small Intestine. Hence, a temporary mild *Ague* or malaise may be experienced.

Psionic Medicine lore states that a medical condition, even when resolved, may leave its effect for years afterwards. It is explained thus: following the resolution of an illness, various and vague adverse symptoms continue because that original illness left a distorting/disturbing pattern recorded within the 'etheric' body. (Thought of as a sort of 'fall out' as from a nuclear explosion). The naming of these distortions: Miasms. These may be cleared, and therefore the 'etheric' body restored, homeopathically. Of course there have to be other methods of restoration such as with the administering of 'Reiki' treatment.

THESE DETOXIFYING AND CLEANSING PROCESSES HAVE VARIOUS NAMES IN VARIOUS THERAPIES:

Healing-crisis   *We use this term in the West and is, self-explanatory - it may occur following several treatments.*

Jei du   *This term is applied in Traditional Chinese Medicine. Meaning: to induce a re-action ultimately for the good.*

Energy-cyst	*.....or release of it, as put forward discreetly by Cranio-sacral Therapy lore. Energy-cyst is the term given to the lodgement of disturbance/distortion in a given area within the energetic and physical bodies following illness or trauma.*
Menken	*This term given in Japanese Shiatsu. It means purposely to induce a re-action to change thereby, a stubborn condition physiologically in a patient causing initial discomfort.*
Ayurvedic Medicine	*There are many cleansing techniques recommended for different types of man suitable for detoxifying his system. Thus, a new beginning will assist a favourable change when subsequently, other remedies are applied. The re-actions to this initial detoxification are usually painful.*

Those who drink alcohol immoderately, and smoke cigarettes, (Cigarettes that, by the way, adversely affects the heart and the kidneys as well as the lungs), those who have been taking prescribed drugs and those who are consuming un-prescribed drugs, others who have suffered epidurals, regular aspirin taking, antibiotics to water tablets (water tablets, sounds so innocent!), The Pill, and more, all are more likely, following alternative medical treatment, to experience a powerful and difficult post-healing re-action. And as a result many of these people may not stay the healing course, it being too painful in its early stages.

It is known that women who suffer from post-natal depression are the ones most likely to have been on a course of prescribed drugs, either before, during, or after pregnancy; and possibly some years well before pregnancy. Substances, prescribed and un-prescribed having a deleterious lasting effect well after the consumption of these substances have ceased.

Goerge Ohsawa (who founded Macro-biotics*) explained it well when he said: 'What has a front has a back'. In other words, do something or take a substance now for allaying a need or quashing pain, and **pay** for that later because the consequences of our actions were not thought-out.

In concluding, I would proffer that post-treatment re-actions indicate that the energetic systems have been primed into greater activity, and stagnation of blood, body fluids, electrical and energetic conduction have been challenged for the good. All life is movement, and when movement ceases there is atrophy. To be positive with patients, explaining re-action processes, and that this may mean for them their particular roadway back to health, should be encouraged.

*The Book of Macrobiotics - Michio Kushi. Japan Publications Inc.

'WHAT HEALING IS': *A PERSONAL VIEW OF THE CONCEPT*

It is a normal human attribute to touch, lay hands-on, to cure a given sickness both in ourselves and in others. The good intention is to change that present 'condition' favourably and to elevate our human spirit also. Our desire is to imbue good 'energy/vigour' into ourselves and into others, as and when.

Left and Right Side Brain:

The statement above indicates a right-side brain bias, and this preferment dominates the character of the practise of Alternative/Complementary Medicine.

Left-side brain, the manifestations of which tend to describe the character of Orthodox Medicine, Orthodox Medicine which is implemented by the employment of: logic, machines, gadgets, chemicals, laboratory tests, x-ray photographs and more, cannot easily reconcile itself with the imagination, spontaneity, ethereality, creativity, and intuition which are products of right-side brain employed in the practice of natural medicine.

Left-side brain manifestations are excellent and proper, for example, when in connection with a person physically traumatised, in that the many extraordinary techniques that are products of left-side brain are brought into play to 'put that person back together again' life may be saved and/or made liveable again.

Moreover, there exists a thousand and one ailments/conditions best suited to an orthodox medical administration, although, these tend to be of a more *horizontal* nature, (bed illness). However, the general ethos of, and the philosophy of this type of medicine applied to most ailments and conditions of a more *vertical* nature, (walking-ill), are in the majority of cases detrimental to the body/mind/spirit.

There is also, even nowadays, often a misplaced sense of awe felt by the recipient of orthodox medical administration towards the doctor, surgeon and consultant.

The body's own healing 'chi' and the 'chi' of the practitioner:

At the outset, in a healing session, an assessment of the depth of a medical condition determines the appropriate *means* and its application to help bolster the body's own corrective power, engendering a more favourable state of balance and, therefore, the ailment is eliminated or at least reduced in its detrimental affect.

In addition, a healthy state of 'chi' is maintained. Indeed the *means* is really the sum total of the 'chi' of the practitioner's will to do, and will to heal, as well as his skill directed towards the patient. Yes, there are many forms of 'chi'. It is above, below, inside and outside!

The bolstering and the support of the body's own fighting capacity may be achieved when the *means* does not interfere with and does not damage the various systems that go to make-up the physiological body and lessen the already depleted state of 'chi'. A *means* that coaxes and encourages, strengthens, empathises, and moves with and not against the pulsating life-force, or 'chi'.

Many wonderful therapies exist (*means*) that do implement the attitudes and ideas discussed above. Bear in mind that Western medical developments of chiropractic, osteopathy, homeopathy, herbal medicine, naturopathy, Alexander and Bowen techniques, craniosacral and other therapies, consciously or unconsciously possess an oriental ethos in their execution as well as in their nature.

Even so, the practitioner is only a vehicle, so to speak, a channel to convey the initial healing impetus. Yet, with his skills he cannot become wholly responsible for results absolute: the patient is shown the way, supported and guided back to a healthy state of balance if the patient desires it, and if the patient decides to change his lifestyle for the betterment of his health!

Good results are obtained when the patient's efforts are concomitant with the therapist's treatments.

ETHOS OF MEDICINE IN THE ORIENTAL AND THE OCCIDENTAL MIND-SET:

Oriental:

Seeing and perceiving a universal picture which includes man's relationship to the world he lives in, his responsibilities to himself and others, seasonal cycles, capacity to be inspired by a clear sky at night, awe at the miracles of life about him - all and everything in relation to personal human experience. An awareness of an intelligent universe whose essence was not created by accident but by design. Comprehending the reason why !?!

This will give the reader an idea of why man's health is affected fundamentally or not

Occidental:

An inability to view the connectivity of things, which on the surface appear unrelated. An inability to appreciate the fundamental laws, which govern and relate man to the cycles of the universe/world about him. Making much of the lesser and not recognising the greater. Separability. Interference.

Interference may not always be misplaced in Western thought and action, conversely, an oriental attitude of doing nothing because it 'will happen anyway' may be an easy cop-out! All these issues have an affect on health - they are the unseen, often hidden reasons!

Most body therapies aid the human prerequisite to soften and unbend somatically, and in our psychological attitude. In this way, inner tension and stress engendered by the vicissitudes of life are anticipated and living remains tolerable, because of the dissipation of these negative forces following 'Zen' treatments.

Some body therapies penetrate into further, deeper strata of body/mind/spirit and actually confront pathological conditions and 'in the round' deal with these conditions with considerable success, healing-wise.

However, just a few therapies are special in that they deal admirably with the first and second items, but also propel the recipient, as well as the giver, upwards to transcend the various levels of the body/mind/spirit into the dimensions of well-being, optimism, peace, acceptance, splendour, and nothingness.

Ideally, the induction of this state of being means the correct treatment be administered for that particular ailment, or non-ailment, and the inner confidence, grace or near grace of the giver be present; all this to support and to nourish the recipient on all levels of body/mind/spirit for this ultimate Zen state as previously described, happily to manifest.

For this Zen state to be experienced, an essential ingredient is engaged, and that is the incomparable human touch, doubtless, the supportive human touch is umbilical in its esoteric nature. This umbilical connection transports us back beyond time and space to the beginning of creation (if there was a beginning!) before man and woman were formed, back to that ethereal, nebulous stage, the stage just before manifestation, the phase whose function was to bathe and to nourish the soul immersed in the upper or inner worlds in beatitude.

Put another way, the loftier, heavenly aspects of a person can be induced to predominate, if only for a while, even so, the effects are profound. Induced deep relaxation, yes, healing for that especial condition, yes, and more, a final blissful oneness with all and everything.

Importantly, this precious spiritual encounter will permeate cellular and molecular structures of the body, from the finest to the coarsest. This surely is the healing absolute we all long-for.

Confidentially, we are receiving this class of vivifying ray, every moment from within and from without, only most of us do not know that we are, fortunately or unfortunately.

SOME <u>SPECULATION</u> ON THE ROUTE OF THE COLON MERIDIAN AS INDICATED IN CHINESE MEDICINE AND WHY IT TAKES THIS CURIOUS COURSE

> *The Large Intestine (Colon) meridian runs from the hand (index finger) into the wrist, forearm, elbow, upper arm, shoulder, neck, mandible and maxillae to the side of the nostril, and is bi-lateral.*

The traditional view of why the colon meridian channel is where it is in the body and especially so in the jaw, is because the mastication of food in the mouth stimulates the colon meridian via the jaw/teeth and alerts the digestive processes to begin. In addition, we could elicit another reason why the colon meridian runs through from fingers, arm, jaw to nostrils by understanding why the *ancients* gave the planet Venus to rule the metal element to which the lung and colon meridians belong, according to Chinese medical theory/philosophy.

Beauty, harmony, tasteful discernment, and grace are Venusian attributes/qualities, and so, if humanity at large did not possess these said characteristics in varying amounts, it [humanity] would be unable to discriminate and to appreciate the value and the quality of many things that have significance. Life would be grey, dull, unexciting, pedestrian, and somewhat ugly.

Some might argue indeed that the present epoch 1990 into 2000 plus, is a period of an eclipse of the Venus principle because there is an absence of elegance, good manners, and decency that are Venusian characteristics at their best. For whatever reason, coarseness and vulgarity are in vogue very strongly - not a good example to our young people!

Tastelessness in all things would be the order of the day, whether in art, music, clothing (fashion), speech, food and goods of all description. Skills of the artisan would be half-heartedly carried-out. All types of products would not be completely finished and therefore shoddy in appearance and inefficient in workings (the purpose is missing): and all this manifesting in our daily life experience.

The Venusian principle in the world and welling-up from our interior being bestows a sense of proportion and balance, beauty in form and of structure; fine curved and angled lines; completion and wholeness. Therefore, the Lady Venus inside and outside of us evaluates and places a value on, <u>and determines the amount of appreciation</u> in all, from the material through to the aesthetic.

Thus, it is with this principle we reject and eject, or accept and assimilate that which we dislike or like accordingly. Suitability for us is at a personal and at a gut level. We absorb, therefore, what is pleasing to us, according to our needs and tastes; we allow the crossing-over, the transmigration, through our internal mental and emotional borders to enjoy that which we are happy to and content to assimilate. This is part of our discriminating and evaluating nature.

With regard to the borders of the more material kind, the body will decide what it needs and what is right for it, and with the material lung and colon (gut) each has a visceral border through which it allows an exchange, a crossing-over, a transmigration, a filtration, an osmosis between oxygen and carbon dioxide with the lung, and with the colon nourishment from its contents, which is then passed-out to be given back to the earth as organic matter etc., etc.,

Noxious smells, the odour of those we know, those we like, and those we love (nostrils), the food we consume, its smell and taste (nostrils, maxillae, mandible). The beauty of form (esp. the human neck and shoulders etc.,). Making love, embracing (arms, forearms). The making of goods, crafts etc., (forearms, hands). The playing of an instrument, writing of letters, articles, information, poetry, and painting (wrist, hands, fingers). These represent some of the relationships between the route of the metal element meridians (which represent the lung and the colon organs), and many departments of life.

Bear in mind also, that inspiration also represents the intake of breath (lung) needed to put meaning into the subjects mentioned above, as well as the affects of these subjects taking the breath away on occasion.

We may now speculate on the possible connection, the reciprocity, and the exchange between our personal characteristic 'space' and the outside world, and on a more organic level the reciprocity and the exchange between our physical borders of the lung and especially so the colon with some elements of creation.

FRIGHTENING STATISTICS

The United Kingdom

Back pain affects most of us.

According to a survey[1] published in 2000 almost half the adult population of the U.K. (49%) report low back pain lasting for at least 24 hours at some time during the year.

In a similar survey carried out 10 years earlier[2] just over one third of the population complained of such back pain.

In 1998[3] almost one in five adults (18%) experienced low back pain for the first time.

It is estimated[4] that up to four out of five people (80%) will experience back pain lasting more than a day at some time during their life.

How long does it last?

- In 1998 in over half of those people who reported back pain the episode lasted for over 4 weeks - affecting 8 million[3] people and in the case of 2.5 million of these the back pain lasted throughout the year.
- Young people are more likely to have brief acute episodes of back pain while chronic pain is more characteristic of older people.

Back pain is a significant drain on our economy

Healthcare costs[1]

- At least 5 million adults consult their GP annually concerning back pain. This leads to costs in primary care of £140.6 million.
- In 1993 it was found that a typical GP practice with 5 GPs and 10,000 patients spends an average of £88,000 a year on patients with back pain.
- NHS physiotherapy costs are estimated at £150.6 million
- 10% of those complaining of back pain visited a complementary practitioner (osteopath, chiropractor, acupuncturist)

Private healthcare costs:

- Physiotherapy: £100.5 million
- Osteopathy: £172.8 million
- Chiropractic: £69.1 million

- **NHS Hospital costs (out patients, accident department, day-care and in-patients) are estimated at over £512 million P/A.**

FRIGHTENING STATISTICS

> - **With more than 190 million working days a year lost as a result of back pain, The Trades Union Congress (TUC) estimates that in 2004, back pain will cost the British Economy more than £8 billion.**

Work related costs

- Back pain is the nation's leading cause of disability, with 1.1 million people disabled by it.[5] By the end of 2004, it is estimated that back pain will have cost the UK benefit system in excess of **£1,900 million per year.**

- Back pain is the number one reason for absenteeism from work.

- Every month, approximately 5% of **people in employment aged between 16 and 64 take time off work with back pain.**

- Back pain disability has risen more quickly over recent years than any other common disability. It rose by 104% from 1986-1992.

- At any one time 430,000 people in the UK are receiving Social Security payments primarily for back pain.[8]

- One in eight (13%) unemployed people say that back pain is the reason they are not working.[3]

Risk factors and causes for low back pain

Back pain is spread fairly evenly across the community in terms of age, sex and geography. The statistics for gender and age distribution are as follows:

Men: 40%
Women: 41%
Ages:
16-24 33%
25-44 36%
45-54 47%
55-64 47%
65+   40%

- Reported back pain is most common in those with skilled manual, partly skilled and unskilled jobs.

- Experts say that it is no longer an affliction restricted to the middle-aged and the elderly. Rising levels of obesity, increased TV viewing and ill-fitting

73

FRIGHTENING STATISTICS

classroom desks mean that the number of children with back trouble has increased dramatically.

- Wendy Emberson, a physiotherapist, said modern lazy lifestyles are contributing to the problem of back pain across all age groups: "Traditionally, back pain first tended to strike people in middle age. It used to tail off among the over-sixties and was rarer still once people reached 70. This picture is changing. Nowadays, physiotherapists are seeing more and more children and young adults with recurrent low back pain - as well as older people," she said. "The human body was not designed to spend long periods of time sitting down - especially not on soft settees and ill-fitting classroom or office furniture. Combine this with obesity, stress, poor diets and inactivity, and it is easy to see why people are . . . more vulnerable to back pain," she added.

- Latest research suggests that while the Midlands and Wales are the worst for back pain in Britain, with 73% of people questioned suffering in the past 12 months, Scots are least likely to suffer back ache, with just 53% experiencing it in the past year. There was little difference in the amount of back pain suffered by people in different social classes.

- Gavin Burt, a spokesman for the the General Osteopathic Council, recently said: "Our lifestyles are a breeding ground for back strains, aches and pains. Even our leisure time could be damaging our health. Slouching in front of the TV for long periods is bad for posture. In an age of inactive children engrossed in the latest computer games, the young are particularly at risk."

- Many women report the root causes for pain in the back are housework and looking after children.

- In a recent survey, nearly a third of women said their back pain was aggravated by vacuuming, 15% said it was brought on by pushing heavy shopping trolleys and 10% said it was caused by dusting or cleaning.

- Dishwashers, lawnmowers and vacuum cleaners were widely criticised for poor design that exacerbated back problems.

- More than three-quarters of mothers with young children blamed the design of prams for causing back strain and 72% believed the same to be true of pushchairs.

- Almost a fifth (16%) of mothers said that reaching for a child seat in a car can start a backache or make it worse.

- Trolleys are a leading cause of back pain, say physiotherapists. Wrestling with uncooperative supermarket trolleys is a leading cause of back pain. The Chartered Society of Physiotherapists (CSP) says that manufacturers must take potential stresses and strains on the spine into account when designing new trolleys.

FRIGHTENING STATISTICS

- A recent poll of public service workers by the country's biggest union Unison found that ambulance workers were most at risk of developing problems with their back.

- Other particularly vulnerable groups included care workers, nurses, porters and domestic staff.

- Physiotherapists say they have seen a surge in the number of men complaining of lower back pain and the trusty wallet is their chief suspect. Experts say men who sit down with their wallets in their back trouser pocket risk damaging key nerves. The condition is becoming so common that it has even been given its own name - hip-pocket syndrome or wallet-neuropathy. The wallet will tilt the pelvis unnaturally, encouraging the pelvis to depart from its natural and healthy horizontal state. This causes skeletal stress, pressure on nerves and thus potentially any number of unpleasant symptoms – sciatica being chief among them.

REFERENCES

1. Palmer K.T, Walsh K, Bendall H, Cooper C & Coggon D Back pain in Britain: comparison of two prevalence surveys at an interval of 10 years B.M.J. 2000 320 1577-1578
2. Walsh K, Cruddes M, & Coggon D. Low Back Pain in eight areas of Britain J. Epidemiol. Comm. Health 1992 46 277-230
3. The Prevalence of Back Pain in Great Britain 1998 Department of Health
4. Maniadakis A., Gray A, The economic burden of back pain in the UK Pain 2000 84 95-103
5. Disability Data from the Labour Force Survey , Labour Market Trends June 1998
6. Klaber Moffett J, Richardson G, Sheldon T.A., Maynard A. Back Pain . Its management & Cost to Society. Centre for Health Economics U. York 1995
7. DSS Analytical Services Division 1999
8. OH guidelines Carter JT, Birrell LN (Editors) 2000. Occupational health guidelines for the management of low back pain at work - principal recommendations. Faculty of Occupational Medicine, London
9. T.U.C. the hidden workplace epidemics 1998
10. The Cost to Britain of Workplace Accidents and Work Related Ill Health 1995/6 Health and Safety Executive 1999
11. Porter J.M. Driving and Musculoskeletal Health The Safety and Health Practitioner Supplement July 1999
12. Helliwell P.S, Smeathers J.E. Driving posture,vibration and Psychosocial factors for back pain in long distance drivers Leeds University 1998
13. University of Surrey quoted in the Safety and Health Practitioner May 1999
14. Musculoskeletal disorders in Supermarket Cashiers Health and Safety Executive 1998
15. Clinical Guidelines for the Management of Acute Low Back Pain Royal College of General Practitioners 1999
16. Balague et al Non Specific Low Back Pain in Children and Adolescents : Risk Factors Eur . Spine Journal 1999 8 429-438
17. Viry P. et al Non specific back pain in Children A search for associated factors in 14 year old school children Revue du Rheumatisme (English edition) 1999 66 381-388

4.2 The USA

- In the USA, it has been reported that 8 out of 10 people will have suffered back pain before they die, and that at any given time there is between 15 and 20 percent of the population is complaining of the problem.

FRIGHTENING STATISTICS

- Low back pain affects 31 million adults at any given time. (Source: American Chronic Pain Association, "Facts About Chronic Pain," Louis Harris and Associates survey for Business and Health Magazine, June 1996.)

- In 1984, a Harris survey revealed that 56 percent of Americans suffered from backaches in the previous year. (Source: R. Sternbach, Survey of pain in the U.S.: The Nuprin Report, Clinical Journal of Pain, 2:4, 1986.)

- Figures show that an estimated 2.5million Americans are totally disabled from back pain alone.

- 13,707,000 people visited a physician's office for primarily back pain in the US 2001 (National Hospital Ambulatory Medical Care Survey: 2001)

- Accounting for the costs of treatment, it is likely that this problem costs the USA over $100 Billion per year. This was 1.5% of the country's GDP in 1998 and was over 3.5% of the total healthcare outlay in the same year.

- In the United States, back pain (alongside the common cold) is the most common problem for which people visit a doctor and is the most common cause of disability under age 45.

- While the total annual cost in the United States for health care and lost productivity is over $100 billion, only 10% of the patients account for 90% of the cost. Thus its management and its impact on American workforce are a major drain on the American economy.

- Absenteeism due to back pain disability are estimated at $40 billion per year. Back pain accounts for about a quarter of the lost or unproductive work in the USA, second only to headaches as the most frequent pain complaint of workers.

- 20% of military discharges in the United States are related to lower back pain.

4.3 Australia

- In Australia, the taxpayer is picking up the bill for nearly a million people claiming Disability Support Pensions, citing a bad back as the cause.

- 20.9% of population self-reported having back pain or disc disorders in Australia 2001 (ABS 2001 National Health Survey, Australia's Health 2004, AIHW)

- 20.7% of female population self-reported having back pain or disc disorders in Australia 2001 (ABS 2001 National Health Survey, Australia's Health 2004, AIHW)

- 21.0% of male population self-reported having back pain or disc disorders in Australia 2001 (ABS 2001 National Health Survey, Australia's Health 2004, AIHW)

- 3,937,000 people self-reported having back pain or disc disorders in Australia 2001 (ABS 2001 National Health Survey, Australia's Health 2004, AIHW)

FRIGHTENING STATISTICS

- 1,944,000 men self-reported having back pain or disc disorders in Australia 2001 (ABS 2001 National Health Survey, Australia's Health 2004, AIHW)

- 1,993,000 women self-reported having back pain or disc disorders in Australia 2001 (ABS 2001 National Health Survey, Australia's Health 2004, AIHW)

4.4 Canada

A national survey carried out in 2003 by the Environs Research Group of Toronto Canada found that:

- Almost two-thirds of Canadian adults suffered from back pain in the past year, and a majority report their pain as moderate to severe.

- The impact of back pain on the daily lives of sufferers ranged from time off work and difficulty concentrating, to restricted family and physical activities, and depression.

- Thirty percent of those surveyed said their pain lasted a month or more including 16 per cent who report back pain that is chronic and continuous. Those who report their back pain as severe are more likely to report that their pain never went away.

- In addition to the human toll, back pain also hurts Canada's economy. Of those who were working at the time they experienced back pain, 15 per cent report losing time off work ranging from a few days (18 per cent) to a month or more (53 per cent). Health Canada estimates that musculo-skeletal disorders, including back pain, cost society a total of $16.4 billion in direct (treatment and rehabilitation) costs and lost productivity.

- The survey found that back pain sufferers turn to a range of different remedies in their search for relief. The most common treatment used to relieve back pain is over-the-counter medication (37 per cent). More than a third of the back pain sufferers surveyed visited either a chiropractor, physiotherapist, massage therapist or family doctor. Fourteen per cent of back pain sufferers did nothing to treat their pain, the most frequent reason being they "thought it would go away".

- Almost nine in ten Canadians (88 per cent) rate back pain as either a "very" (54 per cent) or "somewhat" (34 per cent) important public health issue.

4.5 Denmark

- In 2003, research in Denmark concluded that our increasingly sedentary lifestyles mean that back pain is increasingly affecting the young:

FRIGHTENING STATISTICS

- The study showed that 51% of their 13-16 year olds had reported back pain in the previous year.

4.6 The World

- According to the Bone and Joint Decade (an international body supported by the UN, the World Health Organisation, and the World Bank) over 75% of people in the world will experience low back pain at some stage during their life.

5.0   Industry Trends

The USA Back Products Sector

- A study published in the January 2004 issue of the journal Spine by Duke University researchers says that Americans spend a whopping $27 billion dollars a year on treatments for back pain. Sixty-five million Americans with lower-back pain spent $27 billion last year (2003) on a variety of back pain products and back pain classes.

- The results of a new American study shows that most people prefer drug free care for back pain over taking medications. The survey, conducted by the I/H/R Research Group, a full service market research firm that includes experienced health care managers, interviewed 800 American adults nationwide in the Spring of this year (2004).

  The survey, commissioned by the American Chiropractic Association, showed that more than 80 percent of chronic back pain sufferers surveyed would prefer to avoid the use of medication to treat their ailments. However, a majority of those surveyed were taking either narcotics, muscle relaxants or over-the-counter medications to deal with their pain.

Canadian Back Products Sector

- Canadian consumers spent $21.5 million on back pain products in 1999.

TESTIMONIALS

Dear Alexander,

Just had to email you to put on record my enormous appreciation for your system of Pelvic Correction, and the BackChamp in particular. Using the BackChamp is now an integral and essential part of my life and has given me the power to maintain a trouble free back. I have been using the Regulator Technique for some ten months now, and am well on the way to a permanent cure for lifelong back problems. The recent introduction of the BackChamp makes this so easy that anyone could incorporate it into even the busiest schedule without any effort.

I have suffered from back problems most of my life, with continual back ache and frequent visit to the osteopath when my back "went", since an initial sporting accident which was put down to the ubiquitous "slipped disc". Your system of Pelvic Correction came as a "eureka" revelation, both explaining why things kept going wrong and, more importantly, providing the means to put things right. Anyone who has suffered from back problems knows how draining and demoralising this is and will appreciate how empowering it feels to be able to take control and do something about it yourself.

The BackChamp is brilliant. The elegance and simplicity of the design should win it an award. It is discreet, compact, portable and incredibly easy to use. It has proved effortless to incorporate its use as a regular part of my daily schedule, and that is saying something for someone with my history of trying many things but never persisting with them!

As a final point, the great strength of Pelvic Correction is that it does not invalidate any other form of treatment that you may benefit from, but will act as a perfect complement. It will allow you to maintain and extend the benefits from these other treatments.

Once again, thank you and congratulations Alexander.

Best Regards,

Martyn Williams
Sandhurst, Berks.

Dear Alexander,

I would like to take this opportunity to thank you for providing me with the "Backchamp". The Backchamp has made it so much easier and more comfortable to carry out my pelvic correction exercises, which I now find I can build into my daily routine with ease.

This simple piece of equipment means that I can consistently ensure that my pelvis is aligned from the comfort of my own home – and has meant dramatic improvements in back pain and posture.

Thank you so much.

Kind regards,

Bill Meehan
Pinner, Middx.

Alexander,

Thanks for seeing me yesterday at such short notice. I mentioned to you how useful I am finding the Backchamp. Your system is a revelation. It really is an excellent method of maintaining a good (and straight) back. The Backchamp is incredibly simple and ensures that when I do the exercise, I am confident that I am doing it correctly. Most importantly I take it everywhere with me. Having it to hand means that it has become a regular part of my daily routine – like brushing my teeth. What a difference it has made to my life.

Thank you so very much.

John Martin
London SW11

Dear Alexander

As you know I have been using your new Backchamp device for some time now in order to re-align the pelvic region. While the old exercises to realign my pelvis certainly worked, I have to say that the Backchamp represents a dramatic improvement – making the whole process so much easier and the exercises even more effective.

When you told me that you were developing a new aid for doing the exercises my engineering background made me very interested. As you know I was a civil and structural engineer before retiring. It is not easy to produce something that is easy and comfortable to use as well as durable and portable. All the signs are that you have done the trick. A great product! Everyone with back pain should have one.

Kind regards

Colin Pugh
Richmond, Surrey

Dear Alexander

Just a quick note to tell you how delighted I am with the Backchamp.

I have been using it regularly now for three weeks and am finding it very helpful in relieving my back pain. I am finding that it really helps to release the tension in my lower back and make it feel more flexible. (The side effect of a flat stomach and better thigh muscles is a great added bonus!)

It really is a terrific help in the battle to keep pain at bay and at last I feel I have more control over my back/disk problem.

Look forward to seeing you soon.

Best wishes
Barbara Levett
Notting Hill Gate, London

Alexander,

Well it finally arrived and I'm delighted to report a success story. Following a hip replacement, I endured a constant and pretty severe pain in my right buttock, which I couldn't identify or wholly understand. It was extremely painful and resisting all efforts to eliminate it.

Two weeks of using the Backchamp - it went on holiday with me to Spain - and the pain has gone!!! My posture has improved greatly and...my young wife tells me I appear 10 years younger !!!!!!!!!!!! HONEST !!!!

Many thanks Alexander

Robert Meldrum
Scotland

Dear Alexander,

On my first visit to see you, I did not think that your system could make such a difference to my life - but it has!

After suffering for 10 years with back and neck pain following a car accident I was willing to try anything.

After a few visits you mentioned about Backchamp - a clever device that would help me align my pelvis and was light and portable. Since then my Backchamp goes everywhere with me - it is the last thing I pack and the first thing I unpack whenever I go anywhere.

I now know that whenever I am feeling uncomfortable all I have to do is use my Backchamp and I will feel so much better. I am now able to go to the gym three or four times a week something I have not been able to do for a very long time, and even after a three hour car journey after just a few exercises the stiffness disappears.

Thank you Mr Barrie for making such a difference.

Amanda Dover
Boreham Wood, Herts.

Dear Alexander,

I forgot to thank you for sending the 'Backchamp' which I received 3 weeks ago. I really feel the device is doing its job. The pelvic correction exercise is so easy now. I am using the Backchamp 4-5 times a day and I am really noticing the difference. So thank you once again.

Kind regards,

Rosie Tyfany
Cheshire

Alexander,

I had suffered from hip and back trouble for more than 10 years before having the good fortune to encounter your work. I had tried everything I could think of with varying degrees of success. Any improvement was only temporary.

The uniqueness of your approach, however, was two fold:

First, you not only correctly diagnosed the misalignment in the pelvic girdle and corrected it, but also found that a discrepancy in leg length contributed to the problem.

Secondly - which was even more important to me, you supplied me with a wonderfully simple and effective device called the "Backchamp". Exercising just a few minutes a day with this device keeps the pelvis aligned correctly. As a result, I am experiencing dramatic improvement to both back and hip pains.

My deep gratitude is due, therefore, to you, Alexander, and your wonderful Backchamp.

Alun Owen
Dyfed, Wales

APOLOGIA FROM ALEXANDER BARRIE

I have been asked many times: "How did this system come into being". I had to reply that I did not consciously set out to invent a particular aspect of medical practice. The System evolved from observation of a vast number of patients who suffered from musculo-skeletal aches and pains and certain other conditions.

I noticed, virtually without exception, that leg length discrepancy was prevalent 98% of the time. Investigating deeper into this, I began to look to the pelvis, as instinct dictated, to ascertain whether the source of different leg lengths derived from the pelvis. Astonished by observing commonplace dislocation of this bony foundation [pelvis], I revelled in the realisation that nine out of every ten cases of pelvic subluxation/dislocation did cause leg length discrepancy as well as other pathological problems.

With all this in mind, I discovered further, the **cause** of many different medical problems a dislocated pelvis sustained, and what was astounding, was that this pelvic conundrum was and is, so very commonplace and that it spawns most spinal problems as well. All this seemed to have been missed by the orthodox medical profession.

It is important to keep in mind that the pelvis actually is the **foundation of the skeletal frame** and, if the pelvis becomes distorted, the bones above and below it easily become disjointed as well, engendering all the usual musculo-skeletal aches and pains we humans suffer.

82

AFTERWORD:

It is truly unfortunate that your Doctor, Consultant and Orthopaedic Surgeon are completely unaware of the System you are now using. Most of our 'Professionals', bless them, prefer not to know about alternative medical developments simultaneously evolving side by side with their own scientific medicine. Scientific medicine which has its wonderful and splendid place but arguably applied inappropriately to many conditions we humans suffer, engendering an even worse medical scenario.

This is largely due to scientific medicine epitomising left-side brain manifestations only. Right-side brain activity yielding an intuitive approach and seeing the 'bigger picture' is almost absent.

Then this will also explain our human habit of organising and reforming our lives via our left-side brain dictates only. By not applying the attributes of intuition, imagination and inspiration of right-side brain, life is giving us rigour, extreme vicissitudes, derangement, negativity and unhappiness manifesting in our daily existence; probably mostly self-made!

We are all only one breath away from living and experiencing the magnificence (within and without) that we are inherently, and, according to our true nature. We would be suffused with this magnificence, by applying an inner as well as an outer universal approach, that is, using all the interior and exterior gifts that God gave us and needed to give us to enable His/Her glory to manifest.

Alexander Barrie is a registered Shiatsu Practitioner and a registered Cranio-sacral Therapist in the United Kingdom. His Practice (Alexalign Clinic) is in Harrow, North West London. He also lectures and gives workshops at home and abroad, particularly with his System of Pelvic Correction. View next page on further biographical note:

Alexander Barrie. Harrow UK. January '05
For one-day workshops on Pelvic Correction contact:
Email: abspc@btinternet.com
Website: www.alexalign.com for more information and to read on
TESTIMONIALS and more.

ESSENTIAL NOTES ABSOLUTE, TO BE BORNE IN MIND WHEN EXECUTING THE 'REGULATOR' TECHNIQUE:

- Keep children away from the Backchamp® device, they may do something unspeakable with it, and, may harm themselves in some way playing with it!

- This device is virtually unbreakable, so you may use any force you wish when working with it

- Though the feet need to be together when applying the ' Regulator ', they may lift apart a little. This does not matter; what matters, is that there is a basic V shape with the lower legs for Part A of this technique, and that the lower legs generally are near to the buttocks – this means the legs are quite folded at the knees

- You may need to correct the pelvis following love-making. The pelvis could even move out-of-kilter, though you may not have been vigorous with your partner, or he/she with you, in the mating process!

- <u>Take your Backchamp® everywhere with you;</u> remember that you may correct your pelvis sitting-down, as long as you are sitting on the outer edge of a chair, and the <u>torso is upright</u>

- If you have not got a Backchamp® device and you are using two objects like a belt and a rolled-up telephone book of sorts to execute the ' Regulator Technique ', then keep them in the car, the office, as well as at the home

- Because we humans turn-over in our sleep many times, it is easy for our pelvises to mis-align. Do what you normally do when you get-up in the morning, and after about 20 minutes you may then carry-out your first Pelvic Correction of the day

- Remember to do your Pelvic Correction immediately following any kind of physical activity, especially so after moving furniture about; and gardening activity

- When pushing around a food trolley in a supermarket, and it wants to go one way and you want to go another way, <u>do not fight the trolley</u> – it is easy for your pelvis to distort giving you discomfort because of the struggle ensuing!

- Sometimes your muscles will lock disallowing the ' Regulator ' Technique to work efficiently, and you will be in pain. You might break-through this muscle lock if you do a one-off Pelvic Correction at a much, much more powerful pace. If this does not work, then you have to visit a chiropractor or osteopath or any other practitioner to re-align the spine, and this will release the pelvis, and you may then carry-on as before with the 'Regulator ' Technique to maintain pelvic and therefore spinal alignment

- You may perform the technique in question, even if your pelvis is straight and aligned - you cannot push the components of the pelvis to distortion

- You may have to execute the 'Regulator Technique' up to 10 times a day on occasion. This depends on what is 'going on' in your life at the time!

84

BIOGRAPHICAL NOTE:

Re-incarnating into this extraordinary world in the middle of the last century and having realised in his latter years that he had been blessed with the inventive and creative spark that many individuals aspire to possess, he was able to develop at least two gifts. This was mainly in the direction of the practice of Medicine, and also in the writing of Music Composition, especially in Latin American classical guitar.

However, the application of specific techniques in his occupation of Alternative Medicine, led him to the creation on the flourishing **Pelvic Correction System** that is helping so many people, in all 'walks of life', to become pain-free with regard to their backs, shoulders, neck, knees and ankles and more.

He has a son by his first marriage. He lives with his present wife in Harrow, England. His Clinic (Alexalign) is also in Harrow.

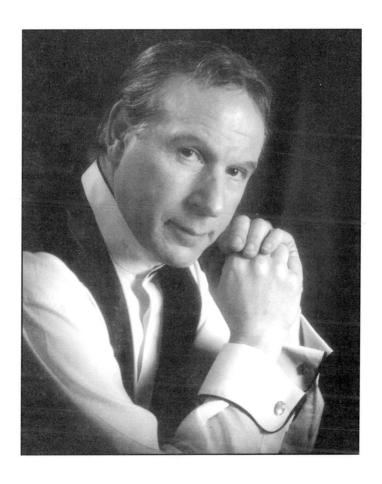

Alexander Barrie

NOTES:

NOTES:

NOTES: